WOMEN IN MEDICINE

WOMEN IN MEDICINE

BY CAROL LOPATE

Published for
The Josiah Macy, Jr. Foundation
by
The Johns Hopkins Press
Baltimore, Maryland

1-15-86

FOREWORD

My interest in utilizing women physicians derived from an international study of medical education in relation to health needs and medical services which I conducted for the Rockefeller Foundation. I was impressed by the large number of women studying medicine in many of the countries that I visited, and I began to gather data on female enrollments. Since then, whenever I talk about women for medicine, I hear the statistic that nearly three-fourths of all physicians in Russia are women. Far more germane to the situation in the United States, however, is the relatively high percentage of women in the countries of Western Europe where the economy and social structure are more like our own. If significant numbers of talented women can be attracted to study medicine in Britain, Scandinavia, and Germany, they can be in the United States.

A variety of factors contribute to the percentage of women entering medicine in different countries. In the countries where essentially mass mobilization was in effect for as long as seven years, women by national necessity entered professional and technical careers. The large numbers of male casualties in two world wars brought widows and daughters to a realization of the need for the long-range security offered by a profession.

Women have been entering medicine in the countries of Eastern Europe in increasing numbers since World War II, and in Bulgaria and Yugoslavia 30 per cent of the medical students are women. The large numbers of female physicians in Russia has been well publicized. These figures (65 to 85 per cent) reflect not only national policy but also personal preference, since medicine in

Russia does not hold the high status that it has in other countries, and the best male students enter other fields of science, technology, commerce, and industry.

In all the countries of Western Europe there are more women in medicine than in the United States. Germany has 30 per cent female graduates—the Netherlands, 20 per cent. In the United Kingdom, at the end of World War II, the University Grants Committee urged that women have greater opportunities to enter medical school, and 25 per cent of the medical students are now women. Where academic salaries are low, in such countries as Great Britain and Israel, a high-income-producing female is an important asset to family stability and an assurance of good educational opportunities for the children. The high figure of 22.5 per cent for women in Israeli medicine is also related to the large number of professional immigrants from Europe to Israel.

In India since World War II, and especially since independence, the figure for women entering medicine has soared. Because of the emphasis that Mahatma Ghandi placed on equal opportunity for women, as well as the easy availability of domestic help, the economic advantage of having two income-producing persons in the family, and the better academic records of women, 35 per cent of all physicians in India are now women. In other partially or entirely Moslem countries, where the tradition of Purdah is still strong, women constitute a less significant proportion: in Pakistan, for instance, only 10 per cent of the medical graduates are women, and in Iran only 6.9 per cent.

Two developed countries which share a low percentage of women physicians with the United States are Spain and Japan. The relatively small figure for women in medicine in Spain, 9.1 per cent, reflects the "duenna" culture of that country—the shielded, almost cloistered life of the daughter—although this is said to be changing in the middle and lower income groups. Strong cultural influences from the Iberian Peninsula have accounted for the relatively modest percentage of women physicians in Latin

America. However, here the trend is upward: recent figures show that in Brazil, 13 per cent, and in Chile, 20 per cent of the medical students are women.

When Japan was under Imperial government, its universities did not accept women, and only a handful of women from families of wealth entered secondary schools—then the emphasis was on domestic arts. However, the number of women students in colleges and universities has quadrupled since 1950, and over 8 per cent of the medical students are now women.

In the light of these statistics, it is distressing that the United States has lagged behind with those countries least willing and able to use their womanpower. Prompted by this state of affairs, and by the acute awareness of the medical shortage in our country, a Macy Conference was convened in October, 1966, at Endicott House in Dedham, Massachusetts. Some thirty educators and physicians were brought together to define the problems of attracting more talented women for the study of medicine, of affording them maximum opportunities for training after medical school, and of keeping them in medical careers once their training has been completed.

The Conference was a lively one, with many valuable suggestions for further action; but the participants were surprised at how little concrete information was available on the subject. The chairman of the Conference, Mary I. Bunting, President of Radcliffe College, suggested that instead of the usual speech-by-speech or word-by-word report that customarily emerges from such a conference, we should aim at an independent study that would synthesize and stimulate discussion. We were fortunate to find Carol Lopate to undertake such a book: we believe that she has hit the target that was set by President Bunting.

There has been so much emotional verbiage written about women in medicine on both sides that it is refreshing to follow the level-headedness which Carol Lopate uses in appraising the situation. This book is neither a polemic nor a recruitment pamphlet. Instead, the author has done what I think is a great deal more unusual: she has inquired into the nature of a woman doctor's life, and communicated the tone and feel of it to us with humor and sympathy. The facts and figures are there, too, but the tensions and rewards of the individuals whom the author has interviewed emerge most sharply. And equally important, along the way one comes to realize the many adjustments—some of them quite small—which could make medical careers more feasible for the wide range of today's intelligent American women.

John Z. Bowers

PREFACE

Do women and medicine have significantly more to offer to each other and to this nation? Advancing knowledge has brought an urgent demand for medical services of many kinds. It has also given women the possibility of many years of professional contribution in addition to fulfilling family responsibilities. Yet the number of women practicing medicine in this country remains very small. Why should this be so? Has medicine little appeal to our young women? Have medical schools discouraged them? Do our standards of professional training present too formidable a barrier? How effective have our women physicians been and how much satisfaction have they found in their careers? What would it take to bring more women into medicine? Would it be worth the effort?

These were the questions that were debated at the Macy Conference on Women for Medicine that led to Carol Lopate's book. They are important questions, with implications that extend far beyond medicine. I am delighted that the book has been written. It provides a sound basis for wide public discussion of these issues, for more realistic career decisions, and for a few critical improvements in the system.

There is no question about the need for more well-trained physicians. Each year hundreds of hospital internships and residency positions go unfilled and, of those taken, a large percentage are held by foreign-trained doctors who may have difficulty understanding either the patients or the professional staff with whom they work. Even people with education and means often have trouble finding good medical care when they need it. Those less advantaged feel helplessly frustrated and seriously wronged.

Do women have a special contribution to make to this situation, and if so, in what way? The problem is far more complicated than most answers, whether pro or con, suggest. Increasing the interest of women in medicine will not of itself bring more physicians into the profession, since the limiting factor is not the number of qualified applicants but the number of places in our medical schools. The average woman physician practices somewhat fewer hours than the average man. Changing the sex ratio in medical school may well add special talents that are in short supply, but there is no reason to believe that it will increase our total resources. This calls for more medical schools and better organization of health care delivery systems.

On the other hand, failure to make good use of those women who do have medical degrees is surely wasteful. The women doctors at the Macy Conference were critical of the rigid requirements of hospitals and specialty boards that made it difficult or sometimes impossible for them to complete their training. Certainly this is an area for imaginative experimentation. Perhaps two well-qualified women sharing an internship over a longer period could provide better service and learn more than some of the interns we now import. Experiments of this kind are being fostered by the Radcliffe Institute in the Boston area. The results look very promising.

This book is intended for young women thinking of medical careers, their advisers (including their families), those who teach them in our schools, our colleges, and our medical schools, the planners who are concerned with medical manpower, and those who are interested in the woman's role in modern society. I hope that it will lead to more informed career decisions and a better understanding of the problems and the potentialities of professional women.

There is no question about the growing need for highly trained talent in this country, or the fact that we have not made good use of feminine intelligence. I believe that a closer examination of this one segment of the population will illuminate some of the problems of medical training and also provide valuable insights toward an understanding of fundamental educational processes.

Today's young women are taking a new look at the professions. This book can be very helpful to them. I particularly hope that it will stimulate interest in new approaches—in medicine and in other fields—that will lead to a more successful integration of women's intellects and energies in our society.

Mary Bunting

ACKNOWLEDGMENTS

This book, by its very nature, has required the interest and energies of more people than I can personally thank. Many, whose
names I do not even know, answered questionnaires sent out by
other researchers; their time and honesty was essential in giving me
pictures of individual women doctors. To the scores of men and
women physicians, medical school deans, educators, and students
whom I myself interviewed, I also owe a large debt of gratitude. It
was their testimony which formed the backbone of the book. I
hope they will be partially recompensed by taking pride in seeing
their words on these pages.

Although this study has diverged in many ways from the original
Macy Conference on Women for Medicine held in October, 1966,
I am indebted to each of the participants. Their ideas were a
springboard for the book, giving me much-needed orientation when
I was still new to the subject. In particular, I must thank Drs.
Helen and Robert Glaser and Ruth Lawrence, who conducted surveys in preparation for the Conference and who gave me free
access to the responses they had collected. President Mary Bunting
and Dean Constance Smith were also extremely helpful, both in
the early stages, with their guidance, and in the end, offering sensitive suggestions about the manuscript.

Drs. Davis Johnson and Edwin Hutchins provided me with a
constant flow of data from the Association of American Medical
Colleges. Dr. Rita Stafford was most generous in lending me her
doctoral dissertation on professional women and the questionnaire
responses which she had used for it. Mrs. Gertrude Conroy, adminis-

trative secretary of the American Medical Women's Association, Dr. Rosa Lee Nemir, its past president, and many other members of that organization opened their doors to me in a most gracious manner.

Three other individuals helped me to the degree that I could not have written the book without them. Dr. John Bowers and Dr. Barbara Rosenfeld, a very special woman doctor, lent their constant encouragement and strength. Above all, however, I owe gratitude to my husband, Phillip Lopate, who went over draft after draft with me, sentence by sentence, and who would not put up with second best.

Carol Lopate

New York

CONTENTS

LIST OF TABLES

LIST OF APPENDICES

WOMEN IN MEDICINE

I

THE ENTRANCE OF AMERICAN WOMEN INTO MEDICINE

The Opening of Medical Training to Women

Throughout the early periods of United States history, it was the common occurrence for American women to work during their adult lives. In pioneer days, they were needed on the farms and in the shops, and often worked side by side with the men. Medical care was frequently the responsibility of the wife or mother. A number of women became famous throughout the colonies for their skill in midwifery: the tombstone of one New England midwife states that she delivered 2,000 babies in her day without mishap. In the 1720's, several women went to Europe to study midwifery, since there were no institutions for medicine in America at that time. The first American medical school was established at the University of Pennsylvania in 1767, and began the tradition of barring women from a medical degree. At various times in the next century, however, women set up flourishing practices on the basis of knowledge they had gained themselves.

Around the second decade of the nineteenth century women began to be separated from the labor force. The advent of industrialization, and the concentration of life around urban centers which came with it, tended to produce a division between the places where men worked and the homes in which women were supposed to take care of their families. The outcry against the squalor of the factories led to their being considered places unfit for women. The sentiment at the time, that industrial plants increased the ugliness of a locality, and the justified fear of poor sanitation,[1] persuaded

[1] It is interesting to note that when women did become involved in medicine, it was because of their concern for public health and sanitation problems. The first chair of Hygiene in the United States was established at the Woman's Medical College of the New York Infirmary.

builders to locate residential areas at a distance from the working centers whenever possible. Reinforcing this separation of the sexes was Victorian morality, which in large part came about because of the attempt to establish some shield of decency within the new order of industrialism, and which fostered the image of women as precious, angelic, and pedestaled objects who would do best to master the arts of homemaking and child-rearing. The very slogan, "A woman's place is in the home," grew out of this situation, since at an earlier period there would have been no conflict—a man's "place" had been at home also, as a farmer, or as an artisan who could usually practice in one section of the house.

In addition to their new isolation, some of the products which women traditionally had made at home were now produced by machine; the scope of their functions was dwindling. When the occupation of "housewife," which had for a century been that of a small group of urban middle- and upper-middle-class women, spread to include a sizable portion of the female population, groups of dissatisfied women began to call for increased opportunities.

> The only careers open to an educated woman were writing, for which few of either sex have adequate talent, and teaching. As school boards found out they could hire women for one-half or less of the pay demanded by men, it dawned on them that women were after all the natural teachers of the young. The result was a rapid increase in the number of women teachers after about 1820, both absolutely and in the percentage of all teachers employed. Many leaders of the women's rights movement, many of the country's first women doctors, started out in a teaching career.[2]

Dr. Elizabeth Blackwell (1821–1910), known as America's first woman doctor, was one of the new generation of discontented women.[3] Although another woman received a medical education from an eclectic school at the same time, and might as justly be considered the first, Dr. Blackwell's life and character reveal a great

---

[2] John B. Blake, "Women and medicine in ante-bellum America." *Bull. Hist. Med.* 39, no. 2 (Mar.–Apr., 1965):107.

[3] The following outline of Dr. Blackwell's life is taken primarily from Mary St. John Fancourt, *They Dared To Be Doctors* (London: Longmans, Green, 1965).

deal about the situation at that time and deserve retelling. Her father, an English sugar refiner, had been an abolitionist and dissenter long before emigrating with his family to the United States. There were nine children in the family. The two older girls, Elizabeth and Emily, were in their teens when the Blackwells settled in New York; allowed more than the usual freedom because of their father's liberal outlook, they often went about town alone in the evening to attend political and social meetings. When Mr. Blackwell failed to establish a successful business in New York, he moved the family to Cincinnati. There, the men of the family became involved in the Unitarian Church and the anti-slavery movement, and the girls became friends and followers of Harriet Beecher Stowe, a central force in the political life of Cincinnati.

At their father's death, the Blackwell sisters helped to support the family by establishing a boarding school for girls. But Elizabeth, involved in woman's rights, found herself dissatisfied with teaching as a means of advancing the cause of her sex, and turned the school over to her sister. When a friend mentioned that until that time no women had been admitted into the medical profession, she forthwith decided to become a doctor.

For several years, Miss Blackwell took positions as governess in the homes of physicians so that she could prepare herself for medical school by reading from their libraries. In 1847, she had saved enough money, and began applying to medical schools in New York and Pennsylvania. One after another flatly turned her down; but several letters contained notes suggesting that she might attend if disguised in male clothing. Elizabeth brushed aside the idea, contending that her goal was "a moral crusade . . . a course of justice and common sense, and it must be pursued in the light of day."[4] She was surprised to receive an acceptance in 1847 from

[4] *Ibid.*, p. 27. The first English woman doctor, Dr. James [Miranda] Berry, was discovered to be a woman only after her death in 1865. She had worked all of her life disguised as a man, and had risen to the position of Inspector General of Hospitals for the British Army. See Esther Pohl Lovejoy, *Women Doctors of the World* (New York: Macmillan, 1957), p. 277.

Geneva Medical School, a small chartered medical school in New York (now Hobart College). The circumstances of her admission were strange: the faculty, not wanting to take responsibility for her rejection, had turned the matter over to the students, who—in an uproarious general assembly—voted a unanimous "yes" as a joke. A fellow-student of Elizabeth's and an eye-witness to the event, Dr. Stephen Smith, described his school as follows:

> Being located in the country, the class of students was made up of the sons of farmers, tradesmen and mechanics. A common saying among the people of that vicinity was that a boy who proved unfit for anything else must become a doctor, and the "royal road" to a medical degree was made remarkably easy . . . The rowdyism of the class may be realized when it is stated that the residents in the vicinity endeavored to have the college declared and treated as a public nuisance.[5]

The medical course lasted a little over a year. Throughout, Elizabeth determinedly held herself back from establishing any social relations with the men but insisted that she be admitted to all lectures, including physiology and anatomy. The first woman's rights convention was held during that year at Seneca Falls, only a few miles from Geneva Medical School, but, perhaps because of the pressure she felt to remain as inconspicuous as possible, she did not attend. It is striking that so zealous and opinionated a person as Elizabeth Blackwell was able to suppress this side of her personality during medical training, showing quiet persistence as her principal outward expression. But medicine is a field which has always demanded self-control and which attracts people who are anxious to maintain it; many of the women who have followed in her footsteps are also concerned only with establishing their capacity for work, not their individual views. Between semesters, Miss Blackwell worked at the Almshouse in Philadelphia, where a staff shortage made the directors welcome anyone—even a woman. After graduating at the head of her class, however, she was forced to move to Paris—an important center of clinical medicine—to

[5] *Ibid.*, p. 46.

study obstetrics and gynecology, since she could not find an American hospital which would admit women for training. Even her excellent record failed to set any precedent at Geneva; many years passed before the school accepted another woman.

During the next years, Dr. Blackwell commuted between Europe and the United States, staying wherever she felt most needed in movements emerging for woman's rights. "You know I am not a natural doctor," she wrote a friend, "so I do not confine myself to practice. I am never without some patients, but my thoughts and active interest are chiefly given to some of those moral ends for which I took up the study of medicine."[6] Throughout her later life, Dr. Blackwell's greatest concern was organizing the means for removing obstacles within the field of medicine so that more women could enter it. For a time she worked in England, helping to liberalize the schools there. In 1857, in order to provide a place for women medical students to receive practical training in America, the New York Infirmary for Women and Children was established by Dr. Blackwell, along with her sister Emily, who had received a degree from Cleveland Medical College (now Western Reserve), and a German physician, Dr. Maria Zakrewska. The Infirmary was housed in the slums of the lower East Side and, despite the angry mobs which stormed the building twice when a patient lay dying inside, they managed to treat over 3,000 in the first year and increased their service thereafter. In 1865, the three women founded the Woman's Medical College of the New York Infirmary, so that American women could receive high-quality medical education. Both projects were soon left in the care of her sister and Dr. Zakrewska, however. Much of Elizabeth Blackwell's time was spent writing and giving lectures on the role of women in medicine and other areas. She never married; one historian who studied her correspondence has commented: "Uncertain in her relations with the opposite sex, she looked to a medical career to 'place a strong barrier' between herself and 'all ordinary mar-

[6] Fancourt, *They Dared To Be Doctors*, p. 126.

riage.' "[7] In her later years she became increasingly interested in health and moral chastity and wrote several books on how to stay healthy through such disciplines as diet and exercise.

Most of the women entering the field of medicine in the time of Elizabeth Blackwell were unable to find openings in regular medical institutions. The majority received their training in the schools of the eclectic and homeopathic sects[8] which were generally more liberal towards accepting women students. These groups, while espousing questionable medical doctrines, were at the forefront of many movements at the time: they supported anti-slavery, temperance, health education, and woman's rights.[9] The first medical school to adopt a policy of coeducation, the Central Medical College of New York at Syracuse, was an eclectic institution; it enrolled ninety-two students in its first session in 1849–50, of whom three were women.[10] The National Eclectic Medical Association formally approved coeducation for women in medicine by a resolution in 1855, and in 1870 became the first medical society to accept women for membership.

An alternative to sectarian schools presented itself around the same time. In various cities throughout the country—sometimes for quite different reasons—agitating groups were working to open medical colleges exclusively for women. In the late 1840's, Dr.

[7] Blake, "Women and medicine in ante-bellum America," p. 102.

[8] *Eclecticism* was based on the principle of embracing the widest possible range of views; it stressed the use of indigenous plant remedies. *Homeopathy* featured the idea that diseases or symptoms of diseases are curable by drugs which produce similar pathologic effects on the body, and that the effect of these drugs is heightened by giving infinitesimally small doses. Another movement during this period was *chiropracty*, which attributed disease largely to the improper functioning of the nervous system and advocated treatment by adjusting body structures, especially the spinal column. Electrotherapy and hydrotherapy were also popular, although they never gained the prominence of a sect.

[9] Blake, "Women and medicine in ante-bellum America," p. 117.

[10] Kate Campbell Hurd Mead, *Medical Women in America* (New York: Froben Press, 1933), p. 10.

Samuel Gregory had begun giving public lectures on midwifery in Boston. He was strongly opposed to male doctors practicing obstetrics, as he felt it was both immoral and dangerous to the health of the embarrassed mothers. " 'Male-midwifery,' as he called it, trespassed upon female delicacy, and was a great temptation to immorality, tending to lead women down the paths of prostitution, and inducing young men to go into medicine because of their curiosity about women."[11] During his classes he proposed that an institution be founded to instruct women in medical subjects—midwifery among them. Despite his inability to raise funds, Dr. Gregory enlisted the aid of two practicing Boston physicians and in 1848, began instructions at the Boston Female Medical College, the first institution to teach medical knowledge to women. The college started without even a skeleton to use for anatomy; for the first two years it moved from home to home by invitation of its students.

The Boston Female Medical College never became securely established. While traditionalists attacked it for allowing women to enter medicine, Dr. Gregory alienated himself from both the faculty and his supporters because of his laxity of standards in establishing formal education. Soon after his death, the directors of the school were forced to look outside for help. After being turned down by Harvard in their petition to merge, they eventually joined with the then homeopathic medical department of Boston University, forming a coeducational medical college.

Harvard itself had tried to become coeducational in 1850 when, under Oliver Wendell Holmes, it accepted one woman and three Negro students. In reaction to this burst of liberalism, the students rioted. Although the main protest was against admitting the Negro students, the woman—Miss Harriet Hunt—had to withdraw her application as well; it was not until 1945 that women were finally accepted at Harvard Medical School.

In Philadelphia as early as 1842 there was talk among a group of physicians, several of them Quakers, of establishing a medical

---

[11] Blake, "Women and medicine in ante-bellum America," p. 118.

school for women; and in 1848 three members of the first faculty were teaching preparatory classes to women so that they would have the two years of pre-college required of matriculants for diplomas when the school opened. In the spring of 1850, the school was chartered as the Female Medical College of Pennsylvania, and in the fall, a house was rented in which to hold classes. The total cost of fitting the college amounted to $1,564.72. When the doors opened, forty women applied for admission—eight to work for the degree of M.D., and thirty-two others simply to listen.[12]

In the next few years, an obstacle arose which made the founding of the college easy by comparison. Several county medical societies in Pennsylvania as well as the State Medical Society passed resolutions against the professors and graduates of the woman's medical college—the county societies on the basis that women were unfit for medicine, and the state society on the grounds that "some of the professors are irregular practitioners."[13] The three eclectic members of the staff were asked to resign, but the ban remained. The leaders of the college, headed by Ann Preston—a former graduate and great advocate of woman's rights—battled against their exclusion until the beginning of the Civil War, when, along with many others, the College was forced to close. At the end of the war, it reopened as the Woman's Medical College of Pennsylvania, with Ann Preston as its Dean, and she once again took up the fight for admission to the medical societies. After her death in 1874, the old resolutions were finally rescinded in the county societies, and women were allowed to attend the national conventions.

In the meantime, in 1865, the Woman's Medical College of the New York Infirmary had been established. Its leaders, Elizabeth and Emily Blackwell and Maria Zakrewska, were determined to

[12] Gulielma Fell Alsop, *History of the Woman's Medical College, Philadelphia, Pennsylvania, 1850–1950* (Philadelphia: J. B. Lippincott, 1950), p. 14.
[13] *Ibid.*, p. 64.

make the education at their college of the highest quality: they required entrance examinations ten years before such exams were made compulsory by law, and they established a three-and-a-half-year course with a graded curriculum, when many medical schools were still requiring only two years of five months' instruction each year. A Chair of Hygiene was created, which Elizabeth Blackwell filled. Under her influence a regular sanitary visiting service to the city slums was also instituted; this service was headed by a member of the Infirmary staff, Dr. Rebecca Cole, the second Negro woman to receive a medical degree, and a graduate of Woman's Medical College of Pennsylvania.

In general, the women who graduated from these schools during this period were of middle- or upper-middle-class backgrounds; some had fathers or husbands already in the field and studied it in order to become partners in the family practices. The difficulty of elbowing into the entrepreneurial ring—always a problem for women doctors—was accentuated during this period by an "over production" of physicians[14] which tended to keep the women either in group practice or in salaried positions of hospitals, clinics, and universities. Probably the first study of how women physicians used their medical training was conducted in 1879 by a Boston physician, Dr. James R. Chadwick, who published a follow-up survey on the students attending the Woman's Medical College of the New York Infirmary during its first nine years. Of fifty-three graduates, he found that only nine were married: five of these were the wives of physicians and had gone into practice with their husbands. Three were daughters of physicians; all practiced with their fathers. Four had gone abroad as missionaries. Sixteen were physicians "living-in" at hospitals or women's colleges such as Vassar and Mount Holyoke. Four held positions in hospitals, two by com-

[14] Abraham Flexner, *Medical Education in the United States and Canada*. Carnegie Foundation for the Advancement of Teaching, Bulletin no. 4 (1910): 14. In his report, Flexner pointed to towns which numbered as many as three physicians for a population of 100 or 200 citizens. See *Ibid.*, p. 17.

petitive examination. Seven had gone on to pursue their studies in European universities.[15]

The clients of this first generation of women doctors were, in large part, women and children. From the beginning, women of the slums had welcomed their services; then women of the upper classes began to inquire about becoming patients. Many of them, in their Victorian modesty, had suffered ailments for years rather than consult a male physician. When it became known that women doctors were available with services of high quality, these ladies came out of hiding to have their diseases looked after. Many doctors voluntarily chose to treat women and children. Dr. Elizabeth Garrett, England's first legitimate woman physician, once replied to a gentleman who had written to ask if she would treat him for the gout: "Dear Sir, Gout is very much in my line, gentlemen are not. I advise you to consult Dr. So-and-So."[16]

In 1881, Rachel Bodley, Professor of Chemistry and third Dean of the Woman's Medical College of Pennsylvania, sent questionnaires to the 244 living graduates of the school, asking them the nature of their work, their social and financial status, and "last but by no means least, the influence of the study and practice of medicine upon woman's holiest relations, as wife and mother."[17] Of the 189 respondents to her questionnaire, Dean Bodley found 166 engaged in active practices, most of which were in areas dealing specifically with women: 32 were working predominately in gynecological practice; 23 combined gynecology with obstetrics; and 35 combined gynecology with medicine or surgery; 10 were in obstetrics; 9 combined obstetrics and general medicine. There were 10 who worked predominately in internal medicine; 3 in surgery; 7 combined the two specialties, and 37 were in "general practice without discrimination." The incomes of the women ranged from

[15] James R. Chadwick, *The Study and Practice of Medicine by Women* (New York: A. S. Barnes, 1879), p. 74.

[16] Fancourt, *They Dared To Be Doctors*, p. xi.

[17] Rachel Bodley, "The college story." See Alsop, *History of the Woman's Medical College*, p. 127.

under $1,000 to as much as $15,000–$20,000 annually. The average income was $2,970.30. Among these were 7 professors in the medical colleges in Pennsylvania and New York, and 14 lecturers and instructors on the faculty of the Woman's Medical College and in the Woman's Medical College of Chicago. Of the women who reported, 68 had been admitted to a medical society.[18]

Dean Bodley gave particular attention to a perennial problem: the relationship between marriage and the practice of medicine. She stated:

> As it is concerning the phase of influence suggested by this question [What influence has the study and practice of medicine had upon your domestic relations as wife and mother?] that our critics make their severest comments, so it is the most difficult to present truthfully the impressions made by the answers received . . . I have decided to let the statistics speak for themselves. The answers of the 52 married ladies who respond to this question tabulate as follows: Influence, favorable, 45; not entirely favorable, 6; unfavorable, 1. Eleven unmarried reply to this question after striking out from the line the words 'wife and mother.' Of these, 3 state that the study and practice of medicine have prevented marriage, while a fourth states definitely that she has 'remained single for reasons entirely distinct from her profession.'[19]

Dean Bodley also examined the effect of marriage on the practice of medicine:

> The second particular which attracts our attention is the small number of women who have failed to devote themselves to the practice of medicine after graduating . . . Marriage has not interfered with this work, as theoretically it might be supposed to do. Of the whole number of graduates, 54 married since graduation, 75 were already married when they studied medicine. Of the 54 who have married since graduation, only 5 have desisted from practice on account of marriage. Many have achieved brilliant successes since assuming the duties and responsibilities of married life.[20]

[18] *Ibid.*, pp. 130–32. [19] *Ibid.* [20] *Ibid.*, p. 133.

Under Dean Bodley, the tradition was established of sending graduates of the college to India and the Far East as medical missionaries; women from India and Korea were also helped to come to the college for a medical education. The Association of American Women's Hospitals which was formed in World War I grew out of this tradition of foreign service, and many of its workers were graduates of the college.

*   *   *   *

The American Medical Association, which conducted its first annual meeting in Baltimore in 1846, took on the role of working to improve the general standards of medicine amidst the chaos of various sects and cults during the second half of the nineteenth century. Each new society was considered by the AMA another obstacle to its attempts to unify the field; and so great was its desire to bring under control what seemed to be the continually increasing variety of new approaches, that when the societies for the medical specialties first appeared in the 1860's, the Association tried to legislate against them. In addition to societies formed by the sects and specialties, new groups were being established on geographical, racial, religious-missionary, and sexual lines. The impetus for a Negro organization arose largely as a result of the AMA's own restrictive policy: in 1870—ostensibly on the grounds of lower educational requirements—it debarred the National Medical Society of the District of Columbia, a Negro organization, as well as two Negro hospitals, from representation.[21]

At a meeting of the American Medical Association in Washington in 1868, the question of admitting women doctors came up for the first time. Recognition of all regularly educated and well-qualified physicians was advocated, but when a resolution endorsing qualified women doctors was made, it was discussed at length and then indefinitely postponed. In the 1872 meeting of the Association in Philadelphia, another resolution was presented: that

[21] James G. Burrow, *AMA—Voice of American Medicine* (Baltimore: The Johns Hopkins Press, 1963), p. 6.

"while we admit the right of women to acquire medical education and to practice medicine and surgery in all their departments, we deem the public association of the sexes in our medical schools and at the mixed clinics of our hospitals, as impracticable, unnecessary, and derogatory to the instincts of true modesty in either sex."[22]

Dr. D. W. Yandell, president of the 1872 meeting in Philadelphia, mildly defended the right of women to practice medicine, but limited them to certain specialties. "If young and handsome," he said, "I have no doubt valetudinarians of our sex would look for their morning calls as they might for angel visits, only that they would not have them 'short and far between'." Not wanting to take the responsibility for a stand towards women in medicine, he referred the choice to the public. "If they [the people] want women doctors, such will be found ready to meet the demand. If those now pressing forward in their studies so eagerly, find their services are not wanted, they will take down their signs, get married—if they can—or turn lecturers, or to some more lucrative employment. I hope they will never embarrass us by a personal application for seats in the Association. I could not vote for that."[23] After some discussion, the resolution was postponed indefinitely.

At a meeting of the Association in Philadelphia in 1876, a young physician whom observers reported as quite attractive, Dr. Sarah Hackett Stevenson, came as a delegate from the state of Illinois. She had written only her first initial on the roll call, but when she was recognized, it was moved that the names of all female delegates be referred to the Judicial Council. The motion was laid on the table, and no further progress was made for nearly forty years.

Although the American Medical Association exercised discriminatory practices in the area of membership, it saw correctly the great need for unity and standardization of the field. Because the Association was unable to establish an effective means of enforcing standards of medical education and practice until the first decade

[22] Morris Fishbein, *The History of the American Medical Association, 1847–1947* (Philadelphia: W. B. Saunders, 1947), p. 77.
[23] *Ibid.*

of the twentieth century, the programs of the schools continued to vary widely. For entrance, some required that the applicant pass nothing more than an English test; others demanded the minimum of a B.A. degree. Medical schools also suffered from a lack of uniformity in the subject matter offered, due partially to sectarianism. In addition, the length of time required to get an M.D. degree ranged from one to three years. Although some colleges had laboratories and were affiliated with dispensaries and hospitals, many still lacked either of these facilities for practical teaching. Women in medicine generally fared even worse than the men from the standpoint of medical education.

In 1870, however, two new opportunities arose for women wanting to study medicine. First, the University of Michigan Department of Medicine and Surgery became coeducational, setting a precedent for the scores of proprietary schools which appeared in the United States during the next thirty years. Second, Swiss universities opened their doors to women in 1870; Russian and American women in particular seized the opportunity. Of the 120 Americans who studied medicine in Zurich between 1870 and 1910, 57 were women. By 1910, 1,048 foreigners were enrolled in Swiss medical schools, compared with 648 native-born Swiss: 814 of these foreigners were women from Russia, Germany, and the United States.[24] The same pattern developed in Germany a few years later. As a result of these opportunities, there were 2,432 American women doctors registered in 1880; in 1890, there were 4,557; and by 1900, the number had jumped to 7,387.[25]

In the 1890's, two first-rate medical schools opened as coeducational institutions: The Johns Hopkins University School of Medicine in Baltimore, and Cornell University Medical College in New York. The story behind Johns Hopkins' decision to accept women is simple: an endowment of nearly $500,000 was offered by Dr.

[24] Thomas Reville Bonner, *American Doctors and German Universities* (Lincoln: University of Nebraska Press, 1963), pp. 29–30.
[25] Lovejoy, *Women Doctors of the World*, p. 123.

Elizabeth Garrett Anderson at its inception in 1893, on the condition that it waive any restriction of sex. When the trustees accepted the gift, the medical school became the first in America "of a genuine university type"[26] to open on a coeducational basis. The school set another precedent at its opening by requiring of all entrants a four-year liberal arts education.

Between 1850 and 1895, nineteen medical colleges for women had been established, but by 1900, eleven of them were already disbanded, having served their use. By 1910, only two remained, The Woman's Medical College of Pennsylvania (still in existence), and a homeopathic institution in New York. Part of the reason for the short life of women's medical schools can be explained by the generally rapid turnover of medical schools during this period. The United States and Canada had produced a total of 457 medical schools in the nineteenth century, of which many died after a decade and perhaps fifty were still-born.[27]

Abraham Flexner's report on "Medical Education," sponsored in 1910 by the Carnegie Foundation, was written because of the increased concern for raising the quality of medical training, and worked quickly to eliminate or bring up to par those schools whose standards lagged behind. In a special section devoted to "The Medical Education of Women," Flexner came out against separate medical schools for the sexes. In his opinion:

> . . . large sums, as far as specially available for the medical education of women, would accomplish most if used to develop coeducational institutions, in which their benefits would be shared by men without loss to women students; but, if it must be added, if separate medical schools and hospitals are not to be developed for women, interne privileges must be granted to women graduates on the same terms as to men.[28]

Based on his data on the number of women applying to, accepted at, and graduating from medical schools in the first decade of the twentieth century, Flexner arrived at some conclusions

[26] Flexner, *Medical Education*, p. 12.   [27] *Ibid.*, p. 6.   [28] *Ibid.*, p. 179.

which foreshadowed the paradoxes that have accompanied the issue ever since:

> Medical education is now, in the United States and Canada, open to women upon practically the same terms as men. If all institutions do not receive women, so many do, that no woman desiring an education in medicine is under any disability in finding a school to which she may gain admittance. Her choice is free and varied. She will find schools of every grade accessible: the Johns Hopkins, if she has an academic degree; Cornell, if she has three-fourths of one; Rush and the state universities, if she prefers the combined six-year course; Toronto on the basis of a high school education; Meridian, Mississippi, if she has had no definable education at all.
>
> Now that women are freely admitted to the medical profession, it is clear that they show a decreasing inclination to enter it. More schools in all sections are open to them; fewer attend and fewer graduate. True enough, medical schools generally have shrunk; but as the opportunities of women have increased, not decreased, and within a period during which entrance requirements have, so far as they are concerned, not materially altered, their enrolment should have augmented, if there is any strong demand for women physicians or any strong ungratified desire on the part of women to enter the profession. One or the other of these conditions is lacking—perhaps both.[29]

The Twentieth Century

Two strains can be detected among the women physicians who have emerged in the twentieth century: one, a small but militant group of women who are involved with the goal of equal opportunity, and the other, a much larger segment, who have worked quietly with the status quo, rejoiced when opportunities increased, but have not wanted to identify with any "woman's movement." While the first group has been represented largely by the American Medical Women's Association, the majority of women physicians have purposely tried to merge their identity and interests with

[29] *Ibid.*, pp. 178–79.

those of the male segment of the profession. When professional societies have been available, they have joined them; if none opened their doors, they have remained unaffiliated rather than pressing for admission of their sex.

In 1915, coincidental with the year in which women were finally admitted to the American Medical Association, the smaller but more vocal group established the Medical Women's National Association. (The name was changed in 1919 to the American Medical Women's Association.) This group was interested in recruiting more women into medicine, as well as improving the conditions and image of those already in the profession. As the years went by, it became involved in promoting various medical-social issues: the liberalizing of legislation against birth control during the 1920's, then medical insurance, Medicare, and Medicaid, and most recently, abortion reform. On most issues, it has taken an extremely progressive stance, and might have played a more important role in legislative reforms were it not for its small size. Membership in the organization, however, has never risen to more than one-third of the women physicians in the United States—less than 2 per cent of all physicians. A breakdown of the 1965 enrollment showed that only 27.2 per cent of its members were under 40 years old; 23.6 per cent were between 40 and 49; and 22.8 per cent were 50–59; 8.4 per cent were 60–64, and 18 per cent were 65 and over.[30] The generation gap has led to a mistrust of the organization among young women physicians, who feel that too much time is spent fighting for battles already won. One young female intern who attended a recent AMWA meeting described it wryly: "There was a lot of excitement and swapping of stories about injustices to women doctors during World War I."

It is quite understandable if senior members are proud of the work of the AMWA in gleaning early privileges and organizing groups of women banned from the male service groups. During

[30] American Medical Women's Association files, personal communication, April, 1967.

World War I, the AMWA worked with the Suffrage Association
and the American Red Cross to send women doctors overseas, since
they were excluded from enlistment in the military. (Women contract surgeons were employed during World War I, without com-
missions, but with the salary of a First Lieutenant.)[31] Forming a
group on the same principle as the Scottish Women's Hospitals
and the Women's Hospital Corps of England, they called themselves the American Women's Hospitals. Between World Wars I
and II, the organization became an outlet for women physicians
wishing to help out in Europe, as well as in Turkey and Greece;
with the beginning of the Depression, a contingent was established
to give aid to the severely struck areas in the Appalachian Mountains.

In 1940, in anticipation of the entry of the United States into
the war, 2,000 women were registered for American Women's
Hospitals service by the AMWA subcommittee. After the end of
World War II, the American Women's Hospitals continued to
operate in the Near and Far East, including the Philippines, in
connection with the International Medical Women's Association.
While the majority of American women physicians have had little
relation to the work of the American Medical Women's Association, the International Medical Women's Association or the American Women's Hospitals, these groups have given those interested
the chance to become more directly involved in world health.

The struggle of women physicians to enter World Wars I and II
as commissioned officers provides an example of the kind of hesi-
tant steps which even the most aggressive women doctors have
taken to gain equal representation. In April, 1917, when war was
declared by the United States, the Surgeon General of the Army
sent every physician in the country a form to fill out, stating "his"
willingness to serve. Many women physicians volunteered; all were
politely refused. Angered at being barred from serving their country, a group of West Coast women physicians sent a petition to the

[31] Lovejoy, *Women Doctors of the World*, p. 303.

New York branch of the American Medical Women's Association, requesting that action be taken. Correspondence was conducted with Washington, but the petition was rejected. From World Wars I to II, nothing further was done. At the start of World War II a petition was sent again to Washington, and in 1943, President Roosevelt signed a bill which stated: "That hereafter during the present war, and six months thereafter . . . shall be enacted a measure to provide for the appointment of female physicians and surgeons in the medical corps of the army and navy."[32] Women physicians were commissioned throughout the war, but when it was over, they were barred from the Medical Reserve Corps, a privilege supposedly granted to all who had served. At this point, the leaders of the American Medical Women's Association began to protest in support of women veterans, a maneuver which they suddenly discovered, from the indifferent response of the veterans themselves, had no backing; the women were nicely established in their homes again and unwilling to become involved in a campaign for a right which they weren't even sure they wanted. Most women preferred to identify with their husbands—or their profession—rather than with the cause of their sex.

American women physicians in the twentieth century have not made the numerical progress which their earlier advances might have indicated. With the exception of an upsurge reaching 12 per cent of all medical graduates in the years directly following World War II, they have stayed at a fairly low level, rising only from 4 to 8 per cent of the medical student poprlation.[33] Their entrance into the various phases of medicine once forbidden to them has

[32] Hulda E. Thelander, "Opportunities for medical women," *J. Amer. Med. Wom. Ass.* 1 (9):326. In the academic world, women have lost ground in relation to men since 1930. In the early fifties, women earned under 10 per cent of the doctoral degrees in this country, as compared with approximately 15 per cent in the 1920's; in the 1960's, the percentage increased to only a little over 10 per cent. See Jessie Bernard, *Academic Women* (Cleveland: Meridian, 1966), p. 70.

[33] "Women in medical schools," Association of American Medical Colleges, *Datagrams* 7, no. 8 (February, 1966).

been individual and piecemeal, often the result of one woman's outstanding work or one man's understanding of the situation. The emphasis has been on progress through individuals proving themselves to be worthy, rather than on lobbying to increase their privileges or numbers.

The character of the medical profession itself may have tended to make the women in it lukewarm towards further recruitment measures. In the first place, the high prestige of physicians is connected in the minds of most Americans (including those of women who have gone into medicine) with its being a predominately masculine profession. Those women admitted into its ranks have often been reluctant to give up their minority status, when it might mean lowering their professional prestige at the same time. In the second place, the "emotionally detached" and controlled manner demanded of a physician has been in direct opposition to the rhetoric of a minority movement. Those few women physicians in the twentieth century who have fought for equal rights or special arrangements for their sex have been an embarrassing minority to the larger group. Often the tone of protest has put them off more than the causes themselves, with which they might readily agree.

The American Medical Women's Association has frequently complained that members quit them as soon as they become successful, or that many women doctors benefit from their activities without supporting the organization. However, if the AMWA had been a more intellectually vital center for medical ideas instead of merely a special interest group, it might have attracted the support of the young women and retained the allegiance of the gifted, successful group. The *Journal of the American Medical Women's Association* and its other publications may simply be aimed at a level too low for professionals of such sophisticated scientific interests and training.

The sentiments of those women doctors who have shown reluctance to take group action protesting sexual discrimination may perhaps be summarized by a statement of Dr. Glen Leymaster, President and Dean of Women's Medical College. He writes:

Few will claim that significant limitations on opportunities for women physicians are still in force or that individual women fail to carry their share as well as their male counterparts. The struggle for equal opportunity for women . . . seems to have been won during the last century. That battle having been won, the troops should not be wasted by committing battalions to isolated pockets of resistance worthy of only a squad.[34]

That such pockets of resistance and discrimination exist cannot be denied: they are sometimes so fine and insidious that even a squad is too clumsy to handle them; but the record of the twentieth century has shown that they have a tendency to dissolve by themselves, in the face of the proven worth of women physicians and the national need for doctors.

A woman who was the first graduate of a well-known medical school had applied about the time that World War I was in progress and was told that she would be admitted only because of the military situation and the shortage of men. If things changed and enough men applied, she would be "thrown out." When she got into clinical medicine and the class had a patient with, for example, genito-urinary diseases, she was asked to leave and go to the library for the period. Such restrictions were frequent at that time, but common sense has since triumphed over delicacy, and women medical students are now expected to learn the full curriculum.

It was many years before all medical schools accepted women students. In 1934, 28 per cent had never graduated a woman; in 1939, 19 per cent, and in 1944, 9 per cent were still restricting their enrollment to men.[35] The last holdout was Jefferson Medical College in Philadelphia, which voted to become coeducational in June, 1960.

Although enough medical schools were open to women so that any interested woman could attend, graduate education still posed

[34] Glen R. Leymaster, "An answer, a national center for medical education for women—forecast or fantasy?" *J. Amer. Med. Wom. Ass.* 20, no. 4 (1965):346.

[35] "Women in medicine." *J. Amer. Med. Wom. Ass.* 1, no. 3 (1946):93–94.

an obstacle until the end of World War II. Women found it difficult to obtain internships in hospitals throughout the country. In many cases, while there was no specific prejudice against them, sufficient facilities had not been provided to house both male and female staff. Women were often rejected from internship positions simply because they could not sleep with a male house officer in the same room.

Resistance to women in medicine by others in the profession has, in general, come to take a subtle form, often indistinguishable from "official planning." Since the early days of the twentieth century when Abraham Flexner noted the overcrowding of physicians, such stringent controls have been placed on institutions for medical education that the reverse is now true: the shortage of physicians is considered more acute each year, and the question now revolves around the wisdom of giving a precious place in medical school to a woman who will be less likely to devote every year of her life to the practice of medicine and who may devote herself only part-time to medical practice for a substantial period. Whereas prejudice against women in medicine during the latter half of the nineteenth and the early twentieth centuries was founded on assumptions such as its being "unnatural" to a woman, ill-fitting her delicate state and even the dignity of the male, statements against recruiting women into medicine have more recently been based on lower rates of practice.

Hospitals and medical schools in the United States have generally been slow to accept women physicians on their staffs. Questionnaires sent out by the American Medical Women's Association to all hospitals in the country revealed that in 1934, 43 per cent had never employed a woman doctor, and that ten years later, in 1944, 21 per cent had still never employed one.[36] Although women have been allowed to contribute to the field of academic medicine, their advancement in the university structure has not been judged on the same basis as that of the men. Women have predominated

[36] *Ibid.*

at the lower levels of instructor, senior instructor, and sometimes assistant or associate professor. While more than 1,000 men held the post of department chairman in 78 medical schools in 1965, only 13 women were listed in this high position.[37]

One example of a now-honored woman physician, Dr. Helen Taussig, should be mentioned, since it illustrates the difficulties which women have had in gaining promotions for their efforts. In June, 1945, Dr. Blalock and Dr. Taussig performed their first "blue" baby work at The Johns Hopkins Medical School; the idea was generally known to be Dr. Taussig's, and the surgical accomplishment Dr. Blalock's. This operation was acknowledged throughout the world as a milestone. Dr. Blalock, who was Professor of Surgery at the time, was elected to the National Academy of Sciences that June. Dr. Taussig, on the other hand, remained at her post as Assistant Professor; and it was not until 1959 that she was appointed full Professor of Pediatrics.

While the entranceway into medicine has been smoothed for women, the discrimination that exists against them at the higher levels remains. This may be partially explained by the attitude that their divided loyalties to career and family will keep them from giving the same commitment to an executive post as a man. Dael Wolfe has stated, "The professionally ambitious woman is doubly handicapped in the attainment of her goals, handicapped by the prejudice and competition of men and by the lesser ambitions of most women and the employment policies which take account of that lesser ambition."[38]

During the forties and fifties, that period which Jesse Bernard has called "The Great Withdrawal,"[39] the percentage of women Ph.D.'s dropped drastically, it became fashionable to marry young

[37] "Faculty rank by sex and age for 78 of the U.S. medical schools in operation in 1965–66 academic year." *Faculty Roster* (Association of American Medical Colleges, 1966).

[38] Dael Wolfe, *America's Resources of Specialized Talent* (New York: Harper and Row, 1954), p. 236.

[39] Bernard, *Academic Women*, p. 37.

and to have large families, and the importance of being a good mother was emphasized in the mass media. Many women doctors dropped out or severely curtailed their careers in order to give themselves to their families. Retraining centers are now opening to salvage the professional lives and talents of these women. The current generation of college girls, while disapproving of the wasted potential of their mothers, has tried to hold onto the gains in femininity which were made during the housewife-mother experiment. Women in the 1960's show less inclination to relinquish their careers: there has been a slight decrease in family size and, although the average age of marrying is still young, the figure is rising again. Because of the dual work-load of the majority of women physicians, part-time training and special practice opportunities are a pressing need, thus cutting the ground from under the demands for "equality" of rights and treatment. The new principle most often heard is not equal rights but complementarity. "We are not the same as men, and never will be. We do not want to compete," a doctor-mother wrote, "but only to do our share. Women have something of their own to give to the profession."

II

WHY SOME WOMEN BECOME DOCTORS AND WHY MANY DO NOT

Obstacles to the Decision to Study Medicine

Although studies of aspects influencing motivation towards particular careers have been conducted with increasing frequency in recent years, little has been done concerning the difference in variables which affect men and women. The report of the President's Commission on the Status of Women states:

> Existing studies of education take too little account of sex differences—averages that include performance by men and women often obscure the facts about both. Research agencies should be encouraged to analyze more data by sex. Too little is known about factors affecting motivation in girls, about the effects of economic, ethnic, religious, and regional backgrounds on their aspirations and their learning processes.[1]

The lack of any notable increase in the number of women in medicine during the first half of the twentieth century points to difficulties stemming both from within the profession and from American society as a whole. On the one hand, occupational choice is influenced by professional factors such as the number of vacancies at any one time within the specific occupation; the size of the occupational group; its tendency to expand and its turnover rate; the technical requirements necessary for optimum performance of the occupational tasks; the income, prestige, power, opportunities for advancement, congenial associates, emotional gratification and

---

[1] Margaret Mead and Frances Balgley Kaplan (eds.), *American Women: A Report on the President's Commission on the Status of Women*, and other publications of the Commission (New York: Charles Scribner's Sons, 1965), p. 29.

employment conditions afforded by the occupation, and the information generally disseminated about the occupation—public
knowledge and familiarity with it. On the other hand, the individual's technical qualifications for entering, the value orientations of
the individual, and society's general attitudes (about sexual roles,
race, etc.) play an important part.[2]

In medicine, vacancies within the profession have been limited,
and the size of the occupational group has remained relatively
small, making entrance into it highly competitive. In addition, the
technical requirements for admission into the profession have been
outside the traditionally feminine areas of study. While opportunities for income, prestige and power are great, the "value orientations" of women have been in conflict with this essentially masculine picture of success. Women have been entering a wider area of
study, and the line drawn between what is and what is not acceptable changes constantly, but the fear of stepping outside the
feminine role still exists. A woman physician who entered medical
school in the 1920's was told by a fellow student: "You are not a
man, you are not a woman. You are an unsexed thing, studying
medicine out of morbid curiosity." Another woman who trained
during that period heard a classmate say: "I don't want *my* wife
to know anything I don't teach her."

The attitude toward women professionals has relaxed consider-
ably in the last forty years, but the carry-over still influences high
school girls when they dream of the future. In a paper entitled,
"Why So Few Women Become Engineers, Doctors and Scientists,"
Alice Rossi states:

> Studies and observation show that the contemporary college
> woman persists in wanting a mate more intelligent than herself
> whom she can 'look up to' and vicariously experience life and live
> in his shadow . . . Unless enough women want as a mate an intel-
> lectual peer and a tender comrade in life and work, few will

[2] Peter M. Blau, J. W. Gustod, R. Jessor, R. S. Paines, and R. C. Wil-
cock, "Occupational choice: a conceptual framework," *Industrial Labor
Relations Review* 9 (1956):531.

aspire to or persist in the more demanding professions, and fewer still will make notable contributions to their fields.[3]

In the United States, the common phrase, "my son the doctor," illustrates the parental pride of having a male child enter medicine, as well as the failure to extend this attitude to daughters. Throughout maturation, boys are conditioned to pick themselves interesting, prestigious, and financially rewarding careers, while girls more often are told that if they become good wives and mothers, and perhaps develop some outside skill with which they could earn a living in case something happens to their husbands, they will have done enough.

Many women drift through high school and college, receiving superior grades, perhaps excelling in a particular subject, but hesitating to make a professional commitment which might conflict with their desirability as a marriage partner or their capacity for motherhood. A national study of high school students during the Sputnik crisis in 1957 revealed that 18 per cent of the senior girls of high ability did not plan to enter college, as compared with only 10 per cent of equally competent boys.[4]

In addition, most girls appear to need more rewards for intellectual endeavor than boys in order to feel equally sure of their intelligence. A survey of a national sample of graduating seniors conducted by the National Opinion Research Center in 1961 revealed the following:

> Even women who had participated in honors programs tended to be more conventional, conforming, and cautious than their male counterparts; though better grade-getters, women honors students felt less adequate in their field than the male honors students. . . .

The author concludes:

> Honors teachers can attempt to reassure talented women students

---

[3] See Jacquelyn A. Mattfield and Carol G. Van Aken (eds.), *Women and the Scientific Professions* (Cambridge: The M.I.T. Press, 1965), p. 54.

[4] Charles C. Cole, Jr., *Encouraging Scientific Talent* (New York: College Entrance Examination Board, 1956), chs. 5 and 6.

about their capabilities and encourage them to be less cautious. Honors directors can try to get more faculty women who are models of both femininity and scholarship to teach in the honors program; they can establish honors courses dealing with the problems of women; they can bring their students in contact with women who have successfully combined marriage and career.[5]

Stability rates for girls and boys who thought they wanted to become doctors during the first and middle years of high school also reflect the differential in support that they are given during this crucial period. At the Macy Conference on Women for Medicine, Dr. Helen Astin reported high school data for "Project Talent." In this study, 29 per cent of the boys who had decided to become doctors in the ninth grade still planned on it one year after graduation from high school, while only 9 per cent of the girls had retained their career plans. The two years between the eleventh grade and the first year after graduation show a doubly high stability rate for both groups: 51 per cent of the boys who thought they wanted to be doctors in the eleventh grade still wanted to enter the profession one year after graduating, while 18 per cent of the girls who had wanted to be physicians in the eleventh grade continued to plan to go into medicine.[6] The stability rates for students of both sexes going into medicine, however, are among the highest of any field—the only other professions inspiring such great determination being the clergy and the arts. All three of these occupations assume the character of a calling.

The prospects of marriage and children and the temptations of short-term careers and professions requiring less training which present themselves to girls during these years may account for their greater loss of interest. But the experience and stimulation derived from medicine in this period is also more available to boys than to

[5] Walter D. Weir, "Honors and the liberal arts college," in J. W. Cohen (ed.), *The Superior Student* (New York: McGraw-Hill, 1966), pp. 90–91.

[6] John C. Falanagan and William W. Cooley, *Project Talent. One Year Follow-Up Studies*, Co-operative research project no. 2333 (Pittsburgh: University of Pittsburgh School of Education, 1966), p. 177.

girls. High school boys considering medicine as a career can find summer or after-school jobs in which they watch the physician in patient-care or assist him in the laboratory. Girls, on the other hand, are more often enlisted as "candy stripers," and given the job of helping nurses with temperature readings and meal-tray distribution—experiences which enforce the sexual division between doctor and nurse. The years when the bright girl is in college and forced to make her career decision (unless it is deferred) are also the years when society puts the greatest pressure on her to marry and to raise a family; the pressures to be socially desirable influence, to a great extent, her choice of a major field of study. Dr. Thomas C. Mendenhall, President of Smith College, reports that every few years he asks his women what pecking-order their male friends would give to undergraduate majors for them. It is always the same list: at the top are the "nest-feathering" majors: art, music, and English. Next comes a group of "harmless" majors: history, sociology, and government. At the bottom lie philosophy, mathematics, and the sciences. The enrollment of women in these majors follows somewhat closely the pecking-order which their male friends give them, even in girls' schools where the influence of male opinion may not be as great as in the coeducational universities. As for those who go on to graduate school, Jessie Bernard states:

> The picture that comes through from the various studies is of a bright young woman who has persisted in her studies far beyond other women, happy and at home in the college or university library or laboratories, who finds herself encouraged to continue into graduate work by a professor impressed by her ability, even, perhaps, offered a graduate scholarship or fellowship or assistantship, and who—without relinquishing hopes for marriage—accepts it, not because she purposively and planfully aspires to an academic career but because, at the moment, nothing more attractive offers itself.[7]

It is generally conceded that the United States uses only a frac-

[7] Jessie Bernard, *Academic Women* (New York: Meridian, 1966), pp. 59–60.

tion of its women to their full economic potential, particularly
among the educated classes. Medicine employs a higher percentage
of women than several other professions: over 6 per cent, as compared to 2 per cent in law, and less than 1 per cent in engineering.
Many reasons have been given for the fact that women in other
countries show up in greater numbers in the professional ranks.
It has been pointed out that in Europe family continuity in careers
is stressed, so that a daughter is more encouraged to enter her father's profession than in the United States. In Germany 30 per
cent of the medical graduates are women; in the Netherlands, 20
per cent; and in Great Britain, 25 per cent.[8]

The Soviet Union, which has the largest proportion of women
in medicine (75 per cent), stands in something of a polar relation
to the United States: its official ideological position has always been
to assure equal education and employment opportunities to both
sexes. Because of the male deficit in the population—especially
after the Revolution and World War II—it became an economic
necessity to recruit women in large numbers into the professions,
and medicine was the most popular choice among women. The
successful mobilization of female talent has been accomplished
through full use of mass media

> . . . which extol the accomplishments of women scientists and
> other professional women. The image of the hard-working, pro-
> ductive, and patriotic professional woman is constantly held up
> before the eyes of young girls; as a result, to aspire to follow in
> the footsteps of a famous woman scientist, physician, or engineer
> is perfectly natural for a girl growing up in the Soviet Union
> today.[9]

The enthusiasm of Russian women for careers is borne out by
the observation of the same writer, who reports: "The Soviet
Union has succeeded in creating an atmosphere in which a woman

---

[8] John Bowers, "Women in medicine," *New Eng. J. Med.* 275 (August,
1966):362–65.

[9] Norton Dodge, *Women in the Soviet Economy* (Baltimore: The Johns
Hopkins Press, 1966), pp. 233–34.

feels apologetic if she does not work."[10] Although they comprise 75 per cent of the doctors, they are more often at the medium and lower levels of the profession: only 57 per cent of the directors, deputy directors, and chief physicians of medical establishments are women. This lower level of achievement has been accounted for by the distractions of raising families and performing traditionally female duties. It is interesting to note that the percentage of women in medicine has begun to decline as a result of a drive for greater sexual balance and efficiency, and Russian women are now feeling the squeeze in a policy of admission preferential to men in medical schools and hospitals.[11]

In the United States, where young women have always been discouraged somewhat from entering the field, those few who persist and become physicians must be exceptionally motivated. It is not surprising that in interviews they convey the impression of a rather self-confident group. The reasons for their first interest in medicine are various, and in some cases nearly impossible to trace. The complex of motives which go into a career decision are at times so obscure, so interrelated, or so peculiar a mixture of the best and the worst in a person that they would require a study of his or her entire life. Motivational surveys, except for the most thorough and sensitive, can give us only a crude idea: for instance, a respondent may check "interest in biological sciences," although it was not actually a decisive motive but a helpful adjunct to an earlier interest in medicine. Nevertheless, the responses obtained from women doctors in interviews and surveys point to a common range of incentives and mutual backgrounds.

In comparison with men who become physicians, the background of the women differs not so much in quality as in quantity —that is, the women need more of the "right kind." In a study of first-year medical students in all parts of the United States, 50 per cent of the total group came from large cities or suburbs of large cities; among the women in the sample, however, 60 per cent were

[10] *Ibid.*, p. 53.   [11] *Ibid.*, pp. 244–45.

from large cities or suburbs.[12] While medical students in general come from upper income families (the median family income of medical students in 1963–64 was $9,949, and 14 per cent of these students came from 1 per cent of all U.S. families, with incomes in excess of $25,000 a year),[13] various studies indicate that the women come from even more financially secure backgrounds than men. More female medical students had parent-physicians than did the males in the AAMC sample, and the successful women students had even more physician-parents than did those who made irregular progress. In a study by Rita Stafford of New York professional women, the physician group represented the highest socio-economic background. "More than half came from homes which functioned above the community level (High SES), and two-thirds of the remaining 48 per cent were 'on par' with the community in which they resided." Of this group, 81 per cent of their fathers had been members of either a professional, executive, managerial, or proprietor group; 63 per cent had fathers with college, graduate school, or professional school training; 10 per cent had fathers who were physicians.[14]

Until recently, when medical students were included in government loan programs, it was nearly impossible for a man or woman to enter medical training without family assistance. Individual medical schools have made fellowships available for many years,

[12] Davis G. Johnson and Edwin B. Hutchins. "Doctor or dropout? A study of medical student attrition," *J. Med. Educ.* 41, no. 12 (1966): 1239. Items from this Association of American Medical Colleges study were selected and rerun for women only. Data on successful and unsuccessful women medical students in the following pages are drawn largely from this rerun of both types of women students.

[13] Marion E. Altenderfer and Margaret D. West, *How Medical Students Finance Their Education,* U.S. Department of Health, Education, and Welfare, Public Health Service publication no. 1336 (June, 1965), p. 8.

[14] Rita L. Stafford, "An analysis of consciously recalled motivating factors and subsequent professional involvement for American women in New York state" (unpublished Ph.D. dissertation, School of Education, New York University, 1966), pp. 242–43.

but this is not a widespread practice and only a limited number of hand-picked students in financial need are supported through them. While government loans may have encouraged men from lower economic classes to enter medicine, they have done little to change the economic backgrounds of female medical students. Women are generally reluctant to take loans for higher education because it gives them a "negative dowry," which the birth of children and the ensuing curtailed income will make more difficult to pay back. A woman's entrance into the medical profession is rarely a rise in socio-economic status. Most of the women would have been able to marry into their parents' socio-economic group without entering a profession of their own.

Although the motivation of upward mobility has been relatively unimportant among women, the desire for personal independence appears to be a significant factor. In the AAMC questionnaire which offered twenty reasons for choosing medicine as a career, women ranked "desire for independence" fourth in importance. An "interest in people" and an "interest in science" were tied for first place; "curiosity about the body" was listed second, and the "service motive" was given third place. Interviews with women pre-meds and medical students support this ranking. Respondents often expressed the desire to be their own bosses. "I wanted to do something where I could work by myself, rather than under another person," said a senior at Woman's Medical College, who had decided to become a doctor when she was eleven years old. It may also be that these women want to retain their socio-economic status through their own merits, rather than through dependence on their husbands.

Often coexisting along with the desire for independence, and easily a part of the same personality, is the need for involvement in an engrossing professional activity. "Doctors love to be busy!" exclaimed one physician, expressing in simplified form this need for an engrossing and demanding occupation. Even a four-year-old child who for the first time receives a night call from the family doctor realizes the demands put on a physician—as well as the respect which is accorded to him or her for this devotion. Although women in medicine average less time in practice than men, their combined home-and-practice commitments often give them fuller schedules.

The image which a girl forms of what she can accomplish while still remaining "feminine" has a great deal to do with the educational and professional attainments of her mother. If she grows up with a mother who felt it necessary to achieve a life of her own in addition to caring for the family, she will be more likely to accept a demanding career and not to feel that her total commitment must lie with her own future family. According to Edwin B. Hutchins, "Where a good model exists for the resolution of conflict between home and career, then it is no doubt much easier for a girl to endeavor to do both."[15] In a study by Ginzberg *et al.*, of women receiving graduate degrees at Columbia University in medicine and academic fields, three-fourths had mothers who had worked at some point in their lives.[16]

The lack of a female model for combining a professional life with marriage and family duties may be an obstacle when a girl tries to combine the two in her own life. The AAMC survey of women dropouts from medical school revealed that more than two-thirds had mothers who were housewives, while among the group of women who made regular progress in medical school only half said that their mothers were housewives.

Table 2–1 shows the educational level of the mothers of women medical students, as compared with the educational level of the mothers of male medical students in the same year. Over 15 per cent of the women had mothers who were professionals, as compared to 5 per cent of the men, and on an average the mothers of the women were better educated.

[15] Edwin B. Hutchins, "Minorities, manpower, and medicine." Division of Education, Association of American Medical Colleges, technical report no. S–663 (Evanston, Ill., 1966), p. 5.

[16] Eli Ginzberg and associates, *Life Styles of Educated Women* (New York: Columbia University Press, 1966), p. 29.

TABLE 2–1. COMPARISON OF FEMALE AND
MALE FIRST-YEAR MEDICAL STUDENTS

Mother's educational level	Women	Men
Professional	15.7	5.5
College graduate (4 years)	19.0	16.5
1–3 years of college	28.1	25.4
High school graduate	17.4	25.4
1–3 years of high school	6.6	10.5
7–9 years of school	7.4	8.5
Less than 7 years of school	4.1	3.5

Source: Edwin B. Hutchins, "Minorities, manpower, and medicine," Division of Education, American Association of Medical Colleges, Technical Report no. S–663 (Evanston, Ill., 1966), Table 4.

When both parents are in medicine, a girl may enjoy a great deal of support in becoming a doctor. A first-year medical student who was the daughter of two pediatricians grew up with a strong sense of community medical service. "I just never thought of becoming anything else," she said. "It seemed to me that medicine was the world." While she reported that her parents had never encouraged her overtly to follow in their footsteps, the atmosphere had been more than congenial to such a decision.

Most women, however, do not slide so naturally into medicine. For them, active encouragement becomes an important factor. In an attempt to discover the source and degree of support which women receive for their career plans, Rita Stafford asked professional women—physicians, lawyers, educational and nursing administrators—to whom they had first verbalized their professional choice. In all these professions, more of the women replied that they had first told their mothers and then their fathers.[17] Whether this is because they were testing their idea out on the mothers before attacking the truly important person, or whether they really

[17] Stafford, "Motivating factors and subsequent professional involvement," p. 258.

expected to receive more support from their mothers, is impossible to tell.

A survey of women college graduates at the University of Chicago (including professionals, working women, and housewives) conducted by Alice Rossi supports the contention that women see their mothers as more congenial to professional achievement than their fathers. But the study shows that both parents are seen as more supportive than the other people in the women's lives. The subjects were given a list of professions—architect, business executive, college professor, doctor, engineer, lawyer, and research scientist—and asked "to indicate which of these professional jobs they disapproved of for women, as well as which jobs various other people in their lives considered inappropriate for women." Most tolerant of women in the professional fields were the women respondents themselves: 68 per cent did not disapprove of women in any of the professions on the list. The next category in tolerance were the mothers, followed by the fathers; then came women of the same age and education, and only then their husbands or closest male friends. The women ranked "men their own age and education" last on the list; only one-third believed that these men would tolerate women in any of the above professions.

Rossi concludes:

> It is most interesting to find that women see their fathers as more tolerant and permissive of women entering the masculine fields than their husbands, for it suggests a difference between the role of father *vis-à-vis* daughter and the role of husband *vis-à-vis* wife. It may be that in his father role, a man is freer to encourage his daughter in her pursuits into law, science, medicine, or even engineering, an encouragement he would not extend to his wife or to a woman as a younger courting man, for he would have had to live with the consequences.[18]

The AAMC survey of women medical students supports Rossi's picture of the encouraging attitude of the father—but shows the

[18] Rossi, "Why so few women become engineers, doctors, and scientists," p. 91.

mother to be lagging. First-year students were asked to identify the degree to which each parent favored their entering medicine, both before and after the actual decision was made. Interestingly, both parents were seen as more supportive once the girl was definite about entering medical school, but the mothers did not appear to be as enthusiastic as the fathers. Table 2–2 summarizes the responses of these students to the question: How did your parents feel about your entering the medical profession? Even this, how-

TABLE 2–2. PARENTS' FEELINGS ABOUT
DAUGHTERS ENTERING MEDICINE

| | Before decision was made | | After decision was made | |
	Father	Mother	Father	Mother
Strongly in favor	31	6	55	31
Slightly in favor	11	30	19	54
Neutral	33	14	11	20
Slightly against	9	36	4	9
Strongly against	6	11	11	10
No answer	10	3	—	4

ever, simplifies the matter: parents may be supportive at one minute and show disapproval at the next. It is likely that the girls, hoping to see their fathers' pride in their accomplishments, took more note of it than they did their mothers' reaction. What is clear, though, is that both parents "came around" once the decision had been made. They may or may not have thought in terms of a career for their daughter, but once the girl had decided to work for a higher degree, they backed her efforts. The conditions for receiving a medical education almost make it necessary for the plan to have family backing—financially if not emotionally—and it is difficult to imagine finances forthcoming without some sort of approval. Thus, it can be said that women medical students as a group enjoy the support of their families in their careers.

Of course, the low rate of women physicians attests to the fact that such family endorsement of a daughter's medical plans is the exception, rather than the general rule. Although girls may be rewarded for good grades, academic success is often conceived of as an end in itself; parents are less likely to encourage a girl who receives an *A* in science to follow her inclination towards a scientific career. A resident physician, for instance, said that she had not even thought of becoming a doctor until her older brother entered graduate school in history. "My father had always wanted him to go into medicine," she remarked. "And when my brother switched to history, I decided to fulfill my father's wish. He's a chemist himself, but he used to speak of how he had wanted to be a doctor." Her wish to please him, however, had backfired somewhat once she was advanced in training: "Then he began to speak very adamantly in favor of the 'pure' sciences."

The commonly passive attitude of parents toward a daughter's vocational future, as well as the ambivalence which still exists in regard to a profession for women, means that there is greater opportunity for motivating factors coming from other sources than parents.

In a 1949 doctoral dissertation, "The Professional Status of Women in Medicine," Josephine Williams reported that while the men in her sample were more influenced in their decision to study medicine by family pressure and their respect for a particular physician, the women were often influenced by a job they had held at some time during adolescence.[19] Gropper and Fitzpatrick stated that women who enter graduate school are more apt to have been influenced by experiences at school than the men who enter.[20]

In this respect, it is interesting to note that although the literature on women in medicine is scant and career material practically nonexistent, women medical students ranked the importance of

[19] Josephine J. Williams, "The professional status of women in medicine" (unpublished Ph.D. dissertation, Department of Sociology, University of Chicago, 1949), p. 84.

[20] George L. Gropper and R. Fitzpatrick, *Who Goes to Graduate School?* (Pittsburgh: American Institute for Research, 1959).

"books or articles about medicine" as far more important in their career decisions than did the men.[21] Seeing the movie *Men in White* motivated one woman physician, who said, "I thought this was the perfect profession, for men or women. It was obviously a very idealized concept of doing good . . ." Other portrayals of the medical profession in books and movies have attracted female medical students with their image of humanitarianism—especially when there is no life-model for them to use. Typically, however, the heroines of films, television, and teen-age books are in the paramedical fields and not in medicine itself. Although books have been written on pioneering women physicians (see Chapter 3), no novel on a woman doctor has played the important role of *Arrowsmith* in attracting men into the field. Neither has there been a feminine parallel to Dr. Kildare on television (not that we need lobby for one!).

Many women also report having been influenced by their own illnesses or those of people within the family. One woman had planned to be a high school teacher until her father had fallen ill and she was brought into close contact with physicians and hospitals. Another reported that she had had very bad acne as a teenager. "As my mother took me from doctor to doctor, I became interested in all the possible ways of treating complexion trouble. I decided I would be a dermatologist when I grew up." Her decision to enter medical school was never connected with any goal but that of being a dermatologist.

The following biographical sketch, related by a pediatric intern, illustrates how family influence and experience may work together to form a career decision. As a high school student, she said, she had been a lifeguard. She loved the job: an attractive girl, she was the only female lifeguard at the pool. When she began college, however, her father put his foot down: she must find a job which was also a training experience—why not work in a nearby hospi-

---

[21] Johnson and Hutchins, "Doctor or dropout?" (See Question 21, as compared to rerun for women students only.)

tal, and stay out of trouble? Her hospital job proved interesting, but she would have returned to her lifeguard duties the next summer had her father not suggested, once again, that she work in the hospital. After the second summer, her appetite was whetted and she began to take pre-medical subjects in her sophomore year at college. By the time of graduation, her father had come around to supporting her medical career plans so fully that he looked with worry on her steady boyfriend as a diversion from homework. When they married in her junior year in medical school two years later, her father's greatest concern was that she complete her medical education.

Interestingly, the women physicians in Stafford's sample indicated common disciplinary backgrounds which coincide quite well with the above picture. When asked to check the degree of discipline exercised during their childhood, they checked unanimously that it had been "essentially firm, but reasonable." Apparently, none had felt it as either "lenient" or "harsh" during their youth. On the other hand, while three-fourths of these same physicians recognized that their parents were influential in encouraging them towards their *educational goals,* and two-thirds believed that both parents were influential in their professional attainment, only 13 per cent stated that their parents had been "a major influence" in their *career selection.*[22] It is likely that the parents of these physicians exercised moral control, influencing their direction by implanting a notion of acceptable behavior patterns without specifying a profession, or else by manipulating them towards medicine in a subtle, unstated fashion.

Obviously, the motivations necessary for going into medicine must be fostered: they do not simply spring up one day. And yet, motivation continues to be treated like the "call from within" and assessed as if it were a quantitative, isolable factor by deans of admissions and the students themselves. Because the field of medi-

[22] Stafford, "Motivating factors and subsequent professional involvement," pp. 276–77.

cine is presently structured for men, it has been argued that if a woman is to succeed—that is, persist throughout the long training, and after that, justify her place in medical school by extensive service—she must be even more highly motivated than her male colleagues. The term has been used frequently with women as a scare-device rather than as a helpful guideline. "My dear, if you're not truly motivated, you should never attempt to go into this!"—many girls have heard this or similar warnings (often from women doctors themselves) and after torturing themselves about whether they were sufficiently motivated, they have bowed out. With better counseling, girls might be helped to follow their interests and not to be intimidated if they feel a less than total commitment to their career choice. Women may never equal the motivation of men in medicine as long as they do not have as great a drive to make money or to be the head of the household, and as long as part of their ego is bound up with having children; but this does not mean that they cannot serve the community as well-trained, well-qualified, humane doctors.

III

CAREER GUIDANCE
IN HIGH SCHOOLS

The Role of the High School Counselor

For some time now there has been concern about the large number of girls who lose their motivation to study medicine during the high school and college years, and the blame for this has most often been placed at the door of their counselors. They are seen as the ones who should have detected the signs of interest, and who should have been encouraging even when social pressure or difficulty with a particular subject made the student turn away into an easier path. In many cases, it is true that the counseling has been lackluster or inadequate. It may be, however, that too much is being demanded of the counselors: in most high schools and colleges they simply do not have the time, the power, or the information to accept a major part of the responsibility for the lifelines of their pupils.

The sophisticated student, in general, feels even in high school that counselors can be used for little more than secretarial help. A bright girl's or boy's disdain for guidance may in part be explained by the fact that counselors have a reputation for being behind the times, both in information and in attitude. As an example, it has been noted that women have moved into mathematic and scientific areas since Sputnik, but that their counselors are of a different generation and have not caught on either to the personalities and capabilities of these girls or to the increasing possibilities of careers in the mathematical and scientific fields. In high school, the ex-physical education or health education teacher is not uncommon as a counselor, and the academically oriented student is quick to dismiss whatever advice is received from this source because of the counselor's conspicuous lack of training in the student's prospective field.

> The report of the President's Commission on the Status of Women maintains: In quality as well as quantity, counseling is at present wholly inadequate. The recommended ratio of full-time guidance staff to secondary school students is 1 to 300; the actual ratio is 1 to 550, with great variation among regions and shortages greatest in low-income areas. Many counselors do not meet recommended standards of either the United States Employment Service or the professional associations in the field. Far too few have had supervised practice in counseling women. Counseling based on obsolete assumptions is routine at best; at worst, it is dangerous.[1]

In large schools, where there are two or more persons in the counseling office, one is usually in charge of vocational guidance while the other handles college placement. It is assumed that for those students continuing their studies, advisors in the colleges will take on the responsibility of career advice. The heavy work burden on those in the high school counseling offices makes it nearly impossible for even the most dedicated counselor to assume more than a few students as pet projects and to guard their potential as something valuable and important.

College placement advisors in high school are naturally involved in the practical business of placing seniors; if they know that a freshman or sophomore is taking the required courses, they generally feel that there is nothing more to do. The unstated policy frequently encountered is that counseling is only needed a little before applications for college must be filled out. Implied in this system of preparing the student for the very next stage of his education—whether it be high school, pre-medical, or medical school counseling—is a deferral of total career information. The student proceeds in semi-blindness, from institution to institution—and in

---

[1] Margaret Mead and Frances Balgley Kaplan (eds.), *American Women: A Report on the President's Commission on the Status of Women,* and other publications of the Commission (New York: Charles Scribner's Sons, 1965), p. 31.

the case of medicine, often with very confused ideas about how long the training will last. Recruitment pamphlets frequently use the expression "nine years from the end of high school" to indicate the time required to become a doctor (i.e., until the completion of internship), thus omitting or hinting only vaguely at the residency which has become a standard part of most medical training.

As an experiment, I asked my 14-year-old niece, who is in the tenth grade of an above-average New York public school, to consult her advisor for information about medicine. She had never spoken to the woman, but she knocked on her office door and after sitting down asked: "I was wondering if you could give me some information about becoming a doctor. I'm very interested in medicine as a career." The woman looked at her narrowly: "What grade are you in?"—"The third term," answered my niece. "Come back in a year or two; I can't be bothered now."—"But I'm really interested," persisted my niece. "I just want to know what I'll have to do . . ."—"Well, if you're dying, I mean, I can pull you out of a class some day and have a chat with you. Write down your name on that sheet of paper." My niece has yet to hear from the advisor's office. Many high school counselors would probably give the same response to any student who expresses a strong career interest at an early age.

In all fairness, although insufficient communication between the various cut-off points of the educational process seems to exist, this is not simply a matter of "buck-passing." It would be difficult—or useless—to give a concrete idea of what residency is like to a high school sophomore. There is, in addition, a fear on the part of some high school counselors of over-counseling. They believe in the value of their profession, of course; but at the same time they try to hold up some rational check to the "college panic" which presses students, parents, and teachers alike into increasingly earlier career strategy. They would prefer to see a child's interests broad and uncommitted, at least until his first sampling of various subjects in the college liberal arts program.

At the Macy Conference on Women for Medicine, a discussion

arose on the merits of early career decisions, and Mrs. Joan Fiss Bishop, director of the Placement Bureau at Wellesley College, took exception to the general agreement on early professional orientations: "From where I sit, I get the implication that there is something good about a student's knowing from the age of six that he or she wants to be a doctor . . . If so, this disturbs me greatly. It suggests that the only people whom we consider desirable for medicine are those that have early direction."

While in many of the academic professions women are said to make career decisions quite late, often drifting into the area through the encouragement of a particular professor,[2] it appears that women physicians show an early decision pattern. This is typical of most students entering scientific careers, because of the greater preparation necessary. The American Association of Medical Colleges study on the background of medical students revealed a median age of sixteen for both sexes "first thinking seriously of becoming a doctor"—around senior year of high school.[3] Rita Stafford asked the women in her sample to check the point in their education at which they had decided to enter their careers: 37 per cent of the physicians reported that their decision had been made prior to high school, while an additional 29 per cent said they had made theirs before entering college.[4] It is clear that most women physicians decide on their careers before experiencing the broadening benefits of a liberal arts education.

In a study of six successive classes of medical students at the University of Pennsylvania, Natalie Rugoff found a correlation between the age of decision among these students and their certainty of having chosen the career that best suited them. Of those students

[2] Jessie Bernard, *Academic Women* (Cleveland: Meridian, 1966), ch. 4.

[3] Davis G. Johnson and Edwin B. Hutchins, "Doctor or dropout? A study of medical school attrition." *J. Med. Educ.* 41, no. 12 (1966):1240.

[4] Rita L. Stafford, "An analysis of consciously recalled motivating factors and subsequent professional involvement for American women in New York state" (unpublished Ph.D. dissertation, School of Education, New York University, 1966), p. 329.

who had decided before fourteen, a far smaller proportion had seriously considered other careers than medicine; and the earlier the decision, the more certain was the student that medicine was "the only career that could really satisfy" him.[5]

On the other hand, even if early deciders are more sure that they have chosen the right career, the age of decision appears to matter little in the student's ability to complete his medical education. According to the attrition study by Johnson and Hutchins, the median age for the career decision of students with regular and irregular progress was about the same—18 to 19. "The major significant difference is in the 26 years of age and over category, in which were found only 3.5 per cent of all the regulars as compared with 6.7 per cent of all the irregulars (including 9.5 per cent of all the academic dropouts)."[6]

Because of this factor, most medical schools do not accept students who are over 25. Since women more than men, however, may defer their decision to study medicine until they are surer of their personalities, or until the home-child situation begins to run smoothly, the Woman's Medical College of Pennsylvania has kept an open-door policy for older students. There, perhaps due to the encouraging atmosphere, the attrition rate among the older women is not noticeably higher than among the younger ones.

* * * *

The importance of counseling during the high school and college years varies in inverse proportion to the stimulation, encouragement, and direction which the students receive at home and in their classes. A high school with an atmosphere of intellectual excellence and competition can often succeed with minimal vocational counseling by its staff, leaving the advisors free to arrange for field trips, clubs, and outside professional speakers. It is probable that this contact with the concrete ideas and personalities of a

[5] Natalie Rugoff, "The decision to study medicine," in R. Merton, J. Reader, and P. Kendall (eds.), *The Student Physician* (Cambridge: Harvard University Press, 1957), pp. 109–30.

[6] Johnson and Hutchins, "Doctor or dropout?" p. 1152.

profession will contribute more to the final decision than any amount of traditional counseling, which can only impart second- or third-hand information.

Bronx High School of Science is a school which accepts boys and girls "possessing good mental capacities and a particular interest in science, mathematics, or related fields." Students from all boroughs of New York City are selected on the basis of an entrance examination which tests general scholastic, language, and arithmetic-reasoning ability. The required science curriculum consists of a year each of general science, biology, chemistry, and physics, three years of mathematics, and a half-year of science-techniques laboratory. Elective courses are offered in advanced chemistry and physics, as well as in such areas as the history and development of science, or advanced clinical laboratory techniques. Students who excel may take college freshman courses in the sciences and mathematics, as well as in history and English. Over 99 per cent of Bronx High School students attend college, and few consider careers which do not require at least a B.A. degree. (Virtually none of the girls, for instance, become nurses.) The counselors at Bronx Science do almost no vocational advising: their main work is placing students in good colleges. A recent check-up, however, showed that more than 70 per cent of the students who graduated in 1958 are now in science or related fields.[7] The stimulation of the curriculum, the middle-class background of most of the children with its emphasis on professional success, and the elite spirit which the students themselves feel, all make vocational counseling somewhat unimportant: once the students enter the intellectual stream, they find it easy to maintain their motivation, with or without the promptings of an advisor. In college, they are ahead in completing their science requirements and can easily become candidates for medical school.

The waste of talent due to insufficient or inadequate counseling becomes obvious in a non-academically oriented high school, where the curriculum is not geared toward college entrance, much less

[7] Publication of the Bronx High School of Science, Bronx, New York.

toward preparation for a highly-trained, scientific profession such as medicine. The scarcity of female as well as male medical students from lower-class and rural areas is not only a result of inadequate finances, but also a lack of stimulation and encouragement in the home and at school, which is not being allayed by sensitive counseling. In a discussion of the Negro woman, for example, The President's Commission reports:

> On the high school level, many guidance counselors themselves need to broaden their concepts of realistic opportunities for the young Negro woman who wants to go to college or who is weighing that possibility. This is particularly true in the newly integrated high schools, where guidance for Negro youth often is based on misconception of the individual's capacities and abilities, and a lack of knowledge of the accomplishments of Negro women and of probable social change.
>
> The attitude of expectancy toward obtaining an education or working in certain occupations is crucial. When families and children have limited hopes as to future vocational possibilities, counselors also may believe that a girl or a boy has no chance for a particular type of job.[8]

Recruiters on the lookout for scientific or medical potential in deprived areas continually come up against a lack of preparation on the part of the students—sometimes not because the facilities do not exist, but simply because no one has urged them to make use of the offered curriculum. Recently, programs which allow talented junior high and high school students to spend a summer in more intellectually stimulating environments have been instituted. The Summer Intervention Program, ABC (A Better Chance), the Carnegie Program for Pre-college Students, and Upward Bound are some examples. However, only a few students can benefit by the programs each year, and even those cannot expect in one three-month period to make up for the losses of the past eight-to-ten school years.

In some notable cases, high school counselors have been able, through their own efforts, to turn out a far higher proportion of

[8] Mead and Kaplan (eds.), *American Women*, p. 224.

academically-oriented students than the school would have had under normal conditions. Margaret Anderson, who describes her experiences in *Children of the South*,[9] is one example of a dedicated guidance counselor who has gone into the homes of disadvantaged students, prodded those with potential into working harder, and insisted that compensatory education be supplied to them when their previous training had not been sufficient. After her high school in Clinton, Tennessee, was desegregated, she became particularly interested in the special problems of the newly admitted Negro students. Mrs. Anderson reports that a significant proportion of the Negro children she encouraged went into service professions (medicine, social welfare, or counseling), having expressed the desire to help their own race in return for the chance they had been given. Another factor which she herself omits might well have been the strong model of their guidance counselor.

There is no absolute, built-in limitation on the effect that a high school counselor (or college advisor, for that matter) can have. An intelligent, energetic counselor who manages an easy rapport with the students can use the position as a wedge to expand the hopes and achievement drives of a significant segment of the school. Much depends on whether the counselor is willing to let his office take on a congenial atmosphere where students can drop in after class for informal talks that may eventually touch on career problems. Those counselors who feel that the school psychologist is there for that purpose, or who make their offices inaccessible to advisees who are not at the proper "helping" stage, may find that the students will overlook them by the time they are ready for college or vocational information.

Medical Counseling Literature and Clubs

A girl who is thinking of becoming a doctor need not only rely on her guidance counselor for information. She can turn to the

[9] Margaret Anderson, *Children of the South* (New York: Farrar, Straus, and Giraux, 1966).

career books and pamphlets which are available in most "young adult's" sections of libraries, or in the vocational guidance office of her school. The literature on medicine as a career is, for the most part, marked by a reserved, balanced tone—as opposed to the runaway zeal of many recruitment programs—and is careful to communicate an idea of the demands and sacrifices of the profession as well as its rewards. Again and again, one finds mention of long hours, truncated family life, rigorous intellectual demands, and special personality requirements. The American Medical Association booklet, *Horizons Unlimited*, gives the following typical list of required personality traits for becoming a physician: intelligence, scientific curiosity, self-discipline, physical and emotional strength, interest in people, objectivity[10]—to which a similar list in *Your Future as a Physician* adds: compassion, pleasing personal appearance, good judgment and insight, and equanimity.[11] It is probable, however, that for the type of person the medical profession hopes to enlist, the emphasis on superhuman combinations of qualities and on sacrifice and hardships represents not a discouragement but a positive attraction. Certain booklets are like tests or obstacle courses which the prospective physician is encouraged subconsciously to complete with pride. At the end of each new burden described is the silent challenge: "It's a hard road, not for the weak. Are you still with us? Well then, let's go on to the next phase." And the chapters end with statements full of vague but assured promises to redeem the sacrifice. "The work of the average physician is difficult to measure in hours, but most physicians will tell you that they love every minute of it," writes Dr. William S. Kalb.[12]

One of the problems of counseling literature in general is that it often reflects a somewhat conservative viewpoint or archaic state

[10] *Horizons Unlimited* (Deerborn, Ill.: American Medical Association, 1966).

[11] William S. Kalb, *Your Future as a Physician* (New York: Richard Rosen Press, 1963), pp. 33–36.

[12] *Ibid.*, p. 28.

of affairs within the profession. There is a desire to present a more static image of medicine than there would be in engineering or aeronautics, for example. While conceding that specialization is here to stay, one author presents a strongly biased case for the general practitioner. He also urges that, "No matter what specialty you choose, you will make a better physician if you have been in general practice for five years or more before beginning a hospital residency in a special field."[13] There have been many proposals in the last ten years for overcoming the G.P. shortage—such as training physicians' assistants or creating a new specialty of general practice—but few would agree that deferring and thus further attenuating the education of those who want to specialize in other areas represents a desirable solution.

A notable exception to this static image of the doctor is the Macmillan Career Book, *Physician*, by Dana W. Atchley,[14] which includes many suggestions for modernizing medicine. Atchley presents not merely the bare outlines of a medical career, but a vivid, personal, and quite specific sense of what it is to be a doctor and research scientists.

Almost every medical career publication of the last six years has had a special section on women in medicine. These sections, usually short and a little tentative, say in effect that there used to be a problem, but now there is not. The authors agree that women represent a large reservoir of talent for medicine which is still untapped, and that they are being welcomed into the profession. Much is made of Elizabeth Blackwell's pioneer struggles and achievements, along with the contributions of Florence Nightingale, Mary Putnam Jacobi and, in the twentieth century, such women as Florence Sabin, Frances Kelsey, and Leona Baumgartner. The tentative note comes from the fact that the proportion of women doctors has not gone up sharply, and there is some doubt in

---

[13] *Ibid.*, p. 87.

[14] Dana W. Atchley, *Physician: Healer and Scientist* (New York: Macmillan, 1961).

the authors' minds about how many women are really wanted by medical schools—as well as how many want to get in. What is usually pointed out is that all medical schools in the United States accept women today, and that "in fact, there is one medical school —the Women's Medical College of Pennsylvania—which accepts only women students."[15]

The American Medical Women's Association has published a few booklets which deal specifically with matters of interest to women thinking of a medical career. As opposed to the brochures geared predominately toward male students, these publications emphasize to women the feasibility of becoming doctors. One of them —*Medicine as a Career for Women*[16]—tries to anticipate and answer some of the reservations that a girl contemplating such a life may feel. A testimonial is given, for instance, by a physician who raised her family while practicing medicine on a full-time basis. The booklet is written intelligently for sensible high school readers, but the cartoon drawings in it are at an unsophisticated, elementary school level: a woman smiles as she carries a doctor's bag, beats a cake-batter, sits at her desk writing notes, dances in an evening gown, hugs her baby, hangs up her shingle, and so on. The discrepancy between the text and illustrations seems to reflect insecurity about the level of intelligence of the audience for whom the publication is intended. Whatever the limitations of the AMWA publications, they are the only brochures actively encouraging girls to go into medicine, and they should be given wider distribution than the organization by itself can afford.

Histories of famous women doctors have been and continue to be written, among which the only truly excellent one which this author has seen is *Florence Sabin: Colorado Woman of the Century*.[17] Some others which also focus on the contributions of women physi-

[15] *Horizons Unlimited*, p. 26.

[16] *Medicine as a Career for Women* (New York: American Medical Women's Association, 1965).

[17] Elinor Bluemel, *Florence Sabin: Colorado Woman of the Century* (Boulder, Colo.: University of Colorado Press, 1959).

cians are *Look to This Day!*[18] (a biography of the early years of Connie Guion), *Women Doctors of the World*,[19] *Bowery to Bellevue*,[20] *Great Women of Medicine*,[21] and *Elizabeth Blackwell.*[22] As one would expect, the writing is generally no better nor worse than most biographies for youthful readers—many of the books are sentimental, idealized, highly partial, with an unquenchable urge to point out all of the subject's "firsts" in medicine. A difficulty with these books is that, although they give an aspiring girl the important support of tradition and may steel her heroic determination, most of them fail to develop a realistic picture of what it is like to be a woman physician today. Interestingly, when female medical students are asked to name the biographical or historical books on medicine which influenced them during their pre-med days, most do not recall having read anything on women physicians. This may be the result of the girls' own bias toward seeing their future career as a "male" profession.

Recent ventures in developing and maintaining students' interest in medicine have been the high school medical career clubs. Before 1950, most of the extracurricular activities for students interested in medicine were organized through biology or science clubs. The generally recognized need for an increase in medical personnel brought about the establishment of several specific professional societies. The first of these were the Future Doctors' Clubs, organized by the Sandia Kiwanis groups in various communities. Much more widespread have been the Future Physicians' Clubs, undertaken in 1960 by the AMA as the recruiting arm of

[18] Nardi Reeder Campion and Rosamond Welfley Stanton, *Look to This Day!* (Boston: Little, Brown, 1965).

[19] Esther Pohl Lovejoy, *Women Doctors of the World* (New York: Macmillan, 1957).

[20] Emily Dunning Barringer, *Bowery to Bellevue* (New York: W. W. Norton, 1950).

[21] Ruth Fox Hume, *Great Women of Medicine* (New York: Random House, 1964).

[22] Elizabeth Baker, *Elizabeth Blackwell* (New York: J. Messner, 1944).

their organization. The goal of the organization is the formation of clubs in every community in the United States, either through local medical societies or groups of students acting with school authorities. It wisely admits paramedical as well as medical aspirants—which is one way of helping to ensure that girls will take part in the activities. The *Ars Medica* Club, a third type, was established by the American Academy of General Practice as part of Project MORE, a comprehensive medical recruitment program. All of these clubs feature the same kinds of activities: field trips, guest lecturers, practice in the labs, training in the use of equipment, volunteer work as doctor's or nurse's aides, and summer hospital jobs whenever possible. They are effective starting points for any concerted future effort to attract more girls into medicine.

IV

COUNSELING PRE-MEDS

The typical female pre-medical student is self-reliant and self-motivating, and remains fairly independent from counseling facilities. Often she has decided by her freshman year that she wants to be a doctor, and from that point on, she investigates the situation for herself. Her main source of information is the body of lore handed down from year to year in her college about which students have been admitted to which medical schools, and what qualities medical school admissions officers are looking for in a candidate. If the girl continues in her determination past freshman year, and if she survives the physics and organic chemistry courses, she may become part of an enclave within the college: the dozen or so girls from all four classes who are living and breathing their future medical careers. This group feeling, more than any other factor, becomes the force behind her persistence to devote herself to her studies when classmates in other majors are going away for long weekends to the neighboring male universities or taking off weekday evenings for parties and movies.

"It's a way of life," a pre-med at Barnard College told me. She was straightening her room as we talked, so as not to take off too much time from her studies. "Even the chemistry majors going to graduate schools don't have to work as hard as we do. But we've got to memorize mountains of material. We know who got in last year, and the grades they had. We talk about it all the time. We don't really think about much else but getting into med school." Whether or not the amount of studying that many of the pre-med girls do is really necessary would be difficult to determine. In any case, their dedication to the work ethic is good preparation for the long years ahead.

The group feeling among these girls is not always mutually protective. Because they feel that they are vying for a select number of places, competition may lead to petty treacheries within the group. I was told of girls who had given others confusing explanations of material to set their already uncertain friends off the track. One pre-med girl said that the boys in her chemistry class were known to put a drop of something in another pre-med's unknown solution so that he could not detect its identity; she thought, though, that the girls stopped short of this kind of aggressiveness. The emphasis on studying often leads to falsifications about how much time has actually been spent preparing a lesson, the object being to trick the competitor into spending less time on hers. Such competition occurs, of course, in fields other than medicine, but the reputation of pre-meds for engaging in it has become notorious among other university departments.

Despite the undercurrent of backbiting, pre-medical students feel they have only each other to turn to. Their common future is the basis for professional clubs or fraternities[1] on most campuses. In many schools, the pre-medical society meets on a loose, irregular basis, with periodic speakers, films, and trips to hospitals. Meetings are open to whomever is interested, and there are usually no membership fees.

Within this context of hard work and self-reliance, counseling personnel can at times feel quite left out. When asked to rank a list

[1] Alpha Lamda Delta functions as a gathering place on many campuses for male pre-medical students with a three-point average or better on a four-point scale. Any objections to this fraternity appear to stem less often from women—who are excluded from it—than from pre-med advisors who, in many instances, have fought against the formation of a chapter on their campuses. The reasons cited are that the activities are too time-consuming, lowering study quality rather than helping it, and that the narrow viewpoint of a professional fraternity reinforces the pre-medical school orientation in students who already have little feeling for the liberal arts ideal. On some campuses, pre-med clubs have been discouraged for much the same reasons.

of twenty factors important in their entrance into medicine, women medical students placed "formal vocational counseling" second to the last, followed only by "radio, movies, TV."[2] Women physicians interviewed for this book all testified that no prior counseling could possibly tell them what the experience would be: you really had to go through it yourself. Some few added, as an afterthought, that a talk or two by a visiting woman M.D. might help, but they were not enthusiastic about the idea. They maintained that one had to be a strong and independent type in order to go into medicine, and that those who planned on it were "not the girls who hang around counseling offices." They themselves had gone to an advisor after their minds had been made up—for purely formal assistance.

This reluctance to solicit guidance may, of course, be the fault of bad counseling services. Medical leaders commonly lay the blame on the pre-medical advisors for the lack of female recruits, accusing them of "painting a false and gloomy picture." In an article on "Women in Health," Dr. Catharine Macfarlane, Professor Emeritus and Vice President of the Board of Woman's Medical College, is quoted as saying, "College vocational counselors are the single most potent force steering women away from medicine. They exaggerate the difficulties, inspire false fears of professional handicaps, advise incorrectly that men are given preference, and indicate that the odds are not worth fighting."[3]

It is again my opinion, however, that these counselors do not have even the destructive force attributed to them. For many reasons, their influence is rather small. In the first place, by the time a girl reaches college age, it is extremely difficult to reconstruct her image of the type of woman she should be. According to Alice Rossi:

> Campaigns aimed at the college-age woman which have as their goal increasing the number of women entering the sciences, en-

[2] Unpublished rerun of AAMC data for women only, from Question 21, Johnson and Hutchins, "Doctor or dropout? A study of medical student attrition," *J. Med. Educ.* 41, no. 12 (1966).

[3] "Women in health," *Medicine at Work* 5, no. 5 (November, 1965): 11–12.

gineering, or medicine can have only very slight success. College freshmen do not shift from fine arts to chemistry, journalism to engineering. Hence, such campaigns can help only the tiny minority of college women already interested and committed to such career goals, to implement their choices. The interests behind their career choice are interests generally disapproved of for girls in our society, so that efforts to increase the number of women scientists and engineers must concentrate on much earlier stages of life and must involve basic changes in the rearing of girls and boys and the social climate surrounding them.[4]

Reports from an array of coeducational, as well as girls' colleges, show that only around one-tenth of the number of women students who declare themselves pre-meds early in the fall term of their freshman year actually complete the pre-medical requirements, take the Medical College Admissions Test, and apply to medical school.[5] The group of survivors relative to those who first declared themselves pre-meds is actually smaller when one realizes that some of the applicants are late deciders, who have come from related fields through the stimulation of course work or other experiences during the undergraduate years.

The high rate of pre-medical attrition, however, is not merely the fault of lackadaisical cheerleading by the counselors. Misplaced initial desire (students come to college with a narrow range of career possibilities, which expands as they begin to take courses like psychology or sociology, unavailable to them in high school), financial difficulties, academic shortcomings, and early marriages play a large part in deterring students from carrying through their career plans. Furthermore, it is impractical, from the counselor's standpoint, to try to keep up mass interest for a narrow admissions

[4] Alice Rossi, "Why so few women become engineers, doctors, and scientists." In Jacquelyn A. Mattfield and Carol G. Van Aken (eds.), *Women and the Scientific Professions* (Cambridge) The M.I.T. Press, 1965), pp. 53–54.

[5] Personal communication with pre-medical advisors at Barnard, Radcliffe, and Hunter Colleges, the University of Maryland, and Howard University (December, 1966).

funnel. The usual and quite realistic course is not to put too much faith in the long list of freshman pre-medical declarants, or to treat it as something of a joke until natural processes have reduced it to a more realistic number.

The style and quantity of counseling varies greatly according to the size of the college, its academic reputation, its attachment to a university or medical school, its contact with other institutions, and the socio-economic background of its students. An advisor at a medium-sized Southern school was asked how he got in touch with his pre-meds. "If I really need one," he said, "I just go out onto the main walk between the science buildings during the break in classes, and pretty soon he's bound to come along." In some cases, however, communications between counselors and students become difficult to arrange, and the advisor is forced to use other channels: bulletin boards, letters placed in student mail boxes, etc. One advisor, after showing the editor of his college newspaper that pre-meds counted for nearly 10 per cent of the students on campus, was able to secure a weekly space discussing common problems, deadlines, and guest speakers. Even this means of contacting students is unreliable, though, depending as it does on the students picking up the paper as they dash from class to class. When a large proportion are commuters, the difficulty is compounded: even if the students are aware of a meeting or conference to attend, job or home responsibilities often force them off-campus immediately after their last class.

In most colleges and universities, pre-medical advising is not in the hands of the counseling offices, but is allocated to one or more professors in the science departments. The theory behind giving them the job is probably that they see the students anyway and grow to know them through contact in classes. Most advisors, though, are simply handed the responsibility, with the compensation that they will be freed from an hour or so a week of teaching —actually not an advantageous time exchange. One pre-med advisor in a women's college estimated that her advisory duties took up to twenty hours per week preparing letters of recommendation.

"I'm a glorified secretary!" she exclaimed. Unless the individual
likes organizing and administrative duties, the difficulties of contacting students can lessen his interest in counseling and send him
back to the more rewarding work of teaching or research.

Some advisors have said quite frankly, "We're in the pure sciences. We don't have any stake in coaxing our students into medicine." This attitude certainly poses obstacles to recruitment. Medical administrators commonly attribute these instances of "passive
resistance" to jealousy on the part of the nonmedical professionals.
A reason sometimes given by the advisors themselves is their pride
in the guaranteed intellectual creativity of their field as compared
with the quantity of rote work in medical training. In any case, a
change of plans from medical school to graduate work around
junior year is doubly encouraged by the numerous financial stipends for the latter which are posted on every bulletin board in the
science departments. In the last several years there has been a tendency in some schools for the top student in chemistry or zoology
to choose a doctoral degree over an M.D., partially because of the
financial benefits of attending graduate school and partially because of the character of medical education today. The Carnegie
Report, "The Crisis in Medical Service and Medical Education,"
spells out some of the problems of medical education which have
begun to filter back to undergraduate students:

> The well-prepared first-year medical students show signs of bore-
> dom and are probably ready to enter medical school at the second-
> year level. Their boredom arises not only from the repetition of
> material with which they are already familiar. In addition, they
> find ordinary medical school teaching inferior to the teaching of
> science in the better undergraduate institutions where learning is
> regarded as an active process for the student—which means in-
> volvement in research and the exercise of intellectual initiative
> rather than a spongelike passivity which seems to be expected in
> many medical schools.[6]

[6] *The Crisis in Medical Services and Medical Education,* report on an
exploratory conference sponsored by the Commonwealth Fund and Carnegie Corporation of New York, Fort Lauderdale, Florida (February,
1966), p. 9.

Discouraging students from applying to medical school is often considered a necessary part of the advisor's function, both to uphold the reputation of the college and to protect the student from the pain of rejection. Every advisor feels obligated to safeguard the reputation of his college and to keep the way open for future applicants: he tries not to recommend students who will either be rejected or, if accepted, forced to drop out for academic reasons. Most keep a silent grade cut-off in mind, below which they say they will not support a candidate. This cut-off point ranges from a 2.6 to a 3.0 average on a four-point scale, according to the advisor's private estimate of the standing of his school.

St. —————— College for Women, a small parochial college in an urban residential neighborhood, with students mainly from lower-middle-class backgrounds in the area, is the kind of institution which has very few pre-medical students. About six freshmen in each class declare themselves interested in medicine, and only one of these usually applies to medical school in senior year. The others are often swayed from their plans by low grades in science courses. The Sister who chairs the chemistry department and is pre-medical advisor remarked that she saw the core of her job as discouraging from medicine those students who did not have good academic records (3.0 or over). She had observed girls who were determined to become doctors despite gentle but repeated warnings that their marks were not good enough, and who, when they were finally rejected from medical school, suffered collapses of confidence or nervous breakdowns. Often these very tenacious and highly motivated students who would not accept the realities of their grades, she noted, were daughters of physicians. While feeling that this extreme disappointment was important to avoid, the Sister remarked: "I wonder whether many of these girls wouldn't have made good doctors. Some of them are very capable and interested in people, but they got C's in their chemistry. We have to discourage them, because we don't think that medical schools will take our girls with C's."

At present, only about one-half of all male and female applicants to medical schools are accepted each year. A three- or four-to-one ratio would simply cause vast, unnecessary disappointment; so, by bald statistics, it would seem that counselors are doing an adequate job and, at times, a merciful one. Perhaps they could encourage more women to go into medicine, but there has been no sincere expression of need on the part of medical schools for an increase in women candidates, and it is unreasonable to expect counselors to join in a recruitment program when there are already far more applicants than admissions. Similarly, any recruitment program which operates during such an imbalance will have to pull some punches.

Counselors in coeducational institutions usually claim that they advise boys and girls without differentiation. Statistics of admissions show the same proportion of women and men applicants to acceptances, so there is no reason for assuming prejudice at the medical school admissions level. It is before senior year, when a student decides to apply, that discouragement of women operates most strongly. It has been reported that there are male advisors who will try to dissuade a girl student from going into medicine because they do not consider it a fit field for women and believe that they are doing a service to the man who will have to live with her. Such advisors are in the minority. However, the fact that women medical students have a 15 per cent dropout rate as compared to 7 per cent for the men[7] gives advisors another reason for being particularly cautious about recommending female candidates. Whatever the causes, only the most hardy women become applicants, and these may be said—somewhat ironically, though in strict truth—not to face prejudice in getting admitted to medical school.[8]

One coeducational institution where women are specifically encouraged to go into medicine is Howard University. "I don't spend much time talking to them, because they don't come to see me," said Dr. Herman Branson, pre-med advisor and head of the physics

---

[7] Johnson and Hutchins, "Doctor or dropout?" p. 1140.

[8] "Women in medical schools," Association of American Medical Colleges, *Datagrams* 7, no. 8 (February, 1966).

department. "But I've been pushing medicine as a profession for girls who can qualify. I take credit for a few girls going to med school. I say, don't worry about the money; if you get in, we'll find you some." In the last five years, women students in Howard Medical School's freshman class have increased from 5 to 25 per cent. The social structure of the Negro family, with women in the dominant position, has encouraged Negro girls to be more aggressive than their white counterparts. At present, more Negro women have attended college and hold college degrees than Negro men.[9] While white women constitute only a little over 6 per cent of all white physicians, Negro women doctors make up nearly 11 per cent of the non-white medical profession.[10]

Communication between the Colleges and Medical Schools

The lack of communication between the medical schools and the pre-med advisors, although lessening, is probably still the most important reason for the caution which many advisors show in their counseling. There is only one publication on which all pre-medical advisors seem to rely, the *Medical School Admission Requirements,* published yearly by the Association of American Medical Colleges. This booklet contains a list of all medical schools and their requirements, of which only a few show any variation. It also includes deadlines for transcript applications, test scores, and final acceptances. Under each school is a tabulation of male and female applicants and acceptances, which gives prospective students an idea of their chances of success. Since most pre-med students memorize this book quite early in college, the advisor is usually put in a position of repeating the information as if it were an army manual.

[9] Margaret Mead and Frances Balgley Kaplan (eds.), *American Women: A Report on the President's Commission on the Status of Women,* and other publications of the Commission (New York: Charles Scribner's Sons, 1965), p. 221.

[10] Negro physicians and other Negro health personnel," a research agenda prepared by the Health Resources Study Center, University of Washington Medical School (1966), p. 5.

Since 1961, a magazine issued by pre-medical students at Columbia College, *Pre-Med*, has gone a long way toward filling a gap which the editors feel "has not only existed in the area related to medicine but to all graduate schools: this gap is the fantastic lack of information available to the college student to help him with his choice of vocational study."[11] The magazine has opened its pages to medical school admissions officers and physicians, setting up a very necessary exchange of information about what is expected of the medical candidate. There are articles dealing with the judgment of a candidate's intellectual and nonintellectual characteristics, special recruitment pieces, and reports by medical students on the hardships of the first year, second year, etc. The emphasis is on what the pre-medical student can do to make himself a more appealing candidate, and how he can adapt once he has been accepted: in this sense, the magazine focuses frankly on the premed's obsession with the magical process of admission, while steering clear of problems in contemporary medicine. (Almost no mention is made of women medical students; there are no female members on the staff, and there have been very few female contributors. A short symposium, *Women in Medicine* appeared however in the Spring, 1965, issue.)

In recent years, the medical schools themselves have made special attempts to better their communication with the undergraduate colleges. The Annual Conference of Admissions Officers of Southeastern Medical Schools, for instance, has extended its guest list to include pre-medical advisors throughout the area. Advisors in the region usually call a meeting of all pre-med advisees before the conference to discover what their students want to know. They come prepared with specific questions and can speak directly to the officer of a medical school where one or more of their students have applied. Upon returning to the colleges, they hold the second and often only other pre-medical function of the year. Advisors

[11] Editorial, "Pre-Med: purpose restated," *Pre-Med* 4, no. 1 (Fall, 1964): 3.

attending these conferences note new respect from their pre-medical students.

It is not uncommon for advisors, particularly those in colleges with a substantial pre-medical program, to take an important part in the medical schools' selection process. In some state universities, where more than 90 per cent of the pre-meds go on to the affiliated medical school, the admissions officer forms a liaison with the pre-medical advisor over the years, and comes to rely on his personal opinion regarding the quality of an applicant. "I'm on the telephone nearly every day to talk with our medical school in Baltimore," said Dean Laffer of the University of Maryland, who advises pre-medical students there.

Such extensive communication does not exist for every advisor, or in every part of the country. Pre-medical counselors in some of the better women's colleges, which send up to 10 per cent of their student body to medical school each year, have often complained of their isolation from the medical schools. They are skipped when admissions officers make their tours of undergraduate campuses. It would seem that initiation by the counselors—either to attend meetings of medical school personnel or to visit the medical colleges themselves—would be one of the best ways to decrease the panic about the standards medical schools really require. The sacrifice of a few days each year to keep in touch with the medical schools would bring about an increased capability and engagement in the job, and result in closer rapport with advisees.

V

WOMEN IN MEN'S SCHOOLS

Admissions

Since 86 out of the 87 present four-year medical schools and all of the two-year institutions accept an average of seven men for every woman student, there is some reason to think of the medical colleges as being "men's schools." In the last twenty years, the preponderance of men, however, has not been the result of a prejudiced admissions policy. In reviewing the number of male and female applicants and acceptances to medical schools, it becomes quite clear that the proportion of those accepted in both sexes is approximately equal. The *Journal of Medical Education* reported in a study of 1964–65 applicants that:

> The 824 women who were accepted represent 48 per cent of the 1,731 who applied. This is almost identical to the acceptance rate of 47 per cent for the 17,437 male applicants. In terms of acceptances per applications filed, however, the women fared somewhat better than the men. Although their 6,764 applications represent 8.0 per cent of all those filed, the 824 women who were accepted constitute 9.1 per cent of all 9,043 individuals offered a place. Expressed in other terms, the women had essentially the same acceptance rate as the men even though they filed an average of only 3.9 applications per women as compared with 4.5 per man.[1]

The consistency with which male and female applicants are accepted in equal proportion throughout the medical schools makes one wonder if the selection is, in fact, made without reference to

[1] Davis G. Johnson, "The study of applicants, 1964–65," *J. Med. Educ.*, 40, no. 11 (1965):1026–27.

sex. Can it be that these schools receive, year after year, exactly the same proportion of excellent male and female candidates?

The selection of one particular school by a successful applicant out of all of his or her acceptances may add a random note to the proportions set up by admissions officers, but even here it has been said that usually the same proportion of women and men will enter their class on the first day as had been accepted the previous spring. A case in which this did not seem to be happening occurred quite recently in an excellent urban medical school. It was after the deadline for turning in the deposit to hold space for the 1967–68 freshman class, and the admissions officer had only received four deposits from women out of a class of 84. Because "it would not look good to have so few women," the Dean was in the position of having to go back through his applications and solicit more women for his school. This, of course, is a selective admissions policy which helps minority groups.[2]

Prejudice against accepting women continues to exist, except that it is directed toward some future point when the "minority group" might begin to apply in greater numbers. Although the ratio of women to men in medical colleges has risen steadily in the

---

[2] Another medical school Dean told the following story. For years he had had in his scholarship fund a small amount of money reserved for a Negro woman. Since—as he said—the fund helped rather than worked against a minority group, the school had kept it even after the state law prohibited such a designation from being made. When an academically qualified, light-skinned Negro girl without any financial backing applied to his school, he granted her the scholarship. Four years later, after having received money from the scholarship throughout her training, she complained to the Dean that when she applied for an internship, she had discovered that the transcript of her record contained the added information that she was a Negro. She was preparing to sue the school. The Dean answered, "You're right. You can sue us. But if you sue us for that, I'll sue you for accepting the scholarship under false pretenses!" This is only one illustration of the tricky business of accepting aid designed for members of minority groups, since it may be used to maintain the person in the very inequality he or she had hoped to escape.

past fifteen years from 5.4 per cent to nearly 8 per cent (only now nearing its postwar high of 9.5 per cent in 1948),[3] school heads are still reluctant to allow a much higher proportion of women students than they have at present. The rationale at each new stage of the slightly rising percentage is that women are needed in medicine to fill salaried jobs or "women's specialties" which the men will be reluctant to accept. (It has been said, for instance, that a woman who goes into public health is nearly always superior to the man who would choose the same position.) But the admissions officers feel that if the proportion of women in medicine increases greatly, the number of practice hours given to communities would be severely cut. "With the predicted shortage of the 1970's"— stated one admissions officer—"we have to produce as many physicians as we can who will guarantee sufficient practice. If we accept a woman, we'd better make sure she will practice after she gets out. This year I had to insist that we accept only the better-than-average women."

Admissions selection is based on a number of factors: academic average, pre-medical training, extra-curricular activities during the college years (including service in hospitals, summer research jobs, etc.), MCAT scores and, in most cases, the interview. In addition, state schools are forced to consider geographic location of their applicants, and almost all medical colleges accept more willingly a student who applies with financial backing than one who will be forced to rely on his medical school and part-time work for support.

Since undergraduate institutions vary in their grading systems and a 90 from one school may equal an 85 from another, it is difficult to make a valid study of the academic averages of those applicants who were accepted and rejected by medical schools. However, a comparison of scores of men and women applicants to the class of 1961–62 on the four parts of the Medical College Admissions Test

[3] "Women in medical schools," Association of American Medical Colleges, *Datagrams* 7, no. 8 (February, 1966).

(MCAT), made by the Association of American Medical Colleges, is reproduced below.

Dr. Edwin B. Hutchins, who compiled Table 5–1, states: "The pattern of higher verbal scores and lower quantitative scores for women is consistent with the results of other national testing pro-

TABLE 5–1. MEDICAL COLLEGE ADMISSIONS
TEST SCORES   (MCAT)

Subtest	Men			Women		
	Accepted	Not accepted	Total	Accepted	Not accepted	Total
Verbal ability	531	466	506	554	505	537
Quantitative ability	541	467	512	512	447	490
Modern society	523	469	502	507	462	491
Science achievement	539	459	508	520	446	494

Source: Edwin B. Hutchins, "Minorities, manpower, and medicine" Division of Education, Association of American Medical Colleges, Technical Report no. S–663 (Evanston, Ill., 1966), Table 2.

grams and not particular in any way to women medical students."[4] It is obvious from these scores that women are not being discriminated against in the area of MCAT achievement; other than the verbal section, the scores of those accepted are consistently (but only slightly) lower than the men's.

In most schools, where interviews are part of the admissions process, another variable is used to judge applicants: that is, the strength of their motivation, or as one of the Deans called it— "their stick-to-itiveness." The underlying theory, no matter what term is used for it, is that this quality should exist more strongly in the female candidates than in their male competitors, who ob-

[4] Edwin B. Hutchins, "Minorities, manpower, and medicine," Division of Education, Association of American Medical Colleges, Technical Report no. S–663 (1966), p. 4.

viously will continue in the profession because they must have family-supporting careers. Most admissions officers freely admit that this quality is nearly impossible to test except over a period of years, but their uneasiness as they sit across from the attractive college student, so obviously suited to marriage and having babies, forces them to ask once again: "What will you do if you get married while in medical school?" The Dean of a well-known private institution offered one of the more sensible and specific questions: "How do you plan to handle two careers at once?" But even this, he realized, could give him little more than perfunctory assurance.

The tradition of such questions has forewarned women applicants, and few are likely to be caught off-guard in their lack of "dedication." Some admissions officers have therefore come to design more tricky inquiries to elicit that elusive quality. "Where do you see yourself fifteen years from now?" the girl may suddenly be asked. On the other hand, the officer may inquire about her plans for babies, *not* wanting to hear that she sees her life as totally dedicated to medicine but instead testing whether she has a "normal" or "abnormal" set of needs and goals. A Dean admitted, "When a very feminine-looking gal comes in, I might wonder if she's fit for medicine." Thus, the girl applicant must play it both ways.

The ability of the woman candidate to convince the admissions officer sitting across from her in the interview that she is feminine but strong, dedicated but healthy in her needs, and intelligent but not boorish or domineering, depends probably in the end on some very basic and nonverbal transactions: did the officer like her, did he feel that he could get along with her in a work situation, or at least that she would not aggravate him?

Dean Robert Glaser of Stanford Medical School and his wife, Dr. Helen Glaser, Assistant Medical Director of the Stanford Children's Convalescent Hospital, conducted a survey of women medical students in preparation for the Macy Conference on Women for Medicine. Several items in the questionnaire dealt with medical school admissions. The women in the sample were

divided as to whether they felt their sex had helped or hindered
their admission to medical school. It should be pointed out, however, that all had been admitted and had partially finished their
training. Summarizing the responses, Dr. Helen Glaser reported:

> Several girls stated that their medical school was actively seeking
> qualified and attractive women students, and that somehow they
> had fit the bill and had been admitted. Along with this went the
> feeling that a more favorable ratio of acceptances of applications
> existed for women than for men. A few stated that as women ap-
> plicants they were more often noticed and remembered by admis-
> sions committees. This was to their advantage. A small group of
> girls indicated that their expression of interest in medicine and
> their sincere motivation and dedication was seen by admissions
> officers as pure and unsullied by society's expectations of them as
> potential wage-earners and family bread-winners. Lastly, a few
> girls felt that their anticipation of difficulties in convincing admis-
> sions committees of their acceptability was taken by them as a
> challenge, and helped them, actually, to prepare more thoroughly
> for the encounter with the committee.

On the other hand, Dr. Glaser reported that the apparent road-
block most frequently encountered by girls was statistical evidence
of the higher dropout rate among women doctors. "One girl from a
tax-supported school emphasized the school's obligation to produce
physicians for the state, and she felt that she could understand the
school's reluctance to gamble on a woman. There was a greater
tendency of girls in state schools to cite this concern of their schools
regarding dropouts and nonpracticing rates."

Finances

The extent to which the financial resources of an applicant play
a part in his chance of acceptance varies greatly from medical
school to medical school. Among the 52 per cent of men and
women who have not gained admission to any medical institution
in the past few years, it is likely that at least some would have
made good medical students but that their need for financial assistance or their plans to work their way through made them less

eligible candidates to admissions officers. "We don't like our students to accumulate a large debt," remarked one Dean. But with limited private backing and an inadequate supply of government loans (even with the Health Professions Amendment of 1965), keeping down debts of medical students can only mean keeping out those applicants who had planned to face heavy debts. The optimistic attitude of some educators—"If you want medicine, go to it, and you'll find a way"—cannot be entirely true at this point in history.

The small percentage of medical students from families in the lower economic classes attests to the fact that not only are they discouraged as applicants but that most do not even reach the stage of applying to medical school. A young woman employed as an assistant in a medical research institute told a common story: she had been a pre-med the first year, but had had to work part-time to support herself through the rest of college. After the second year of struggling—with only an increase in debts—she had switched to language as major, which allowed more free time for employment and a little socializing. "It just became obvious to me then that I'd never be able to afford medical school," she said. After graduation, she had taught languages for a year, but her love for medicine had brought her back to a job in which she could work around patients and doctors.

In a study of the social classes of medical students in four representative schools (two public and two private), Dr. Edwin F. Rosinski states that while 54 per cent of the total United States population is in the two lowest social classes, only 12.4 per cent of the medical students in his sample schools represented these classes. "Where are the exceptional students from these groups?" he asks.[5]

Dr. Rosinski readily admits the bad effect which a low economic background may have on learning, retention, and motivation to-

[5] Edwin F. Rosinski, "Social class of medical students; a look at an untapped pool of possible medical school applicants," *J. Amer. Med. Ass.* 193, no. 95 (1965):97.

ward seeking a higher education; however, he mentions that in two typical state universities about 24 per cent of the undergraduate student body comes from the lowest social classes, or twice as many students as are admitted to medical schools. "Is it not reasonable to assume," he concludes, "that finances play a large role in this disparity?"[6]

An article on "The Financial State of the American Medical Student" includes the following table on nonrefundable grants awarded to medical students, as well as graduate students in the life sciences and in the arts and sciences, during the 1962–63 academic year:

TABLE 5–2.   COMPARISON OF NONREFUNDABLE GRANTS AWARDED TO MEDICAL STUDENTS AND TO GRADUATE STUDENTS, 1962–63

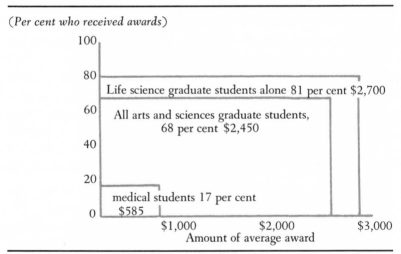

(Per cent who received awards)

Life science graduate students alone 81 per cent $2,700

All arts and sciences graduate students, 68 per cent $2,450

medical students 17 per cent $585

$1,000 $2,000 $3,000
Amount of average award

Source: Joseph Ceithaml, *J. Med Educ.* 40, no. 6 (June, 1965):503. "The financial state of the American medical student."

Although only 17 per cent of all medical students receive nonrefundable awards, and of an average of $585 per year (approximately one-sixth of their total expenses, if they are single), 81 per cent of all students in the life sciences (a natural alternative for a

[6] *Ibid.*

medical school candidate) receive nonrefundable stipends averaging $2,700 annually. The difference in financial backing makes it easy to see the choice that many students with limited resources would be forced to make.

A U.S. Public Health Service study, *How Medical Students Finance Their Education,* reports:

> For all medical students, the largest single source of income was gifts and/or loans from their families, followed by support from their spouses', and their own earnings. Together these sources accounted for 83 per cent of total income. Only 6 per cent of the money came from nonrefundable grants and 10 per cent from loans outside the family.[7]

Women are affected as much, if not more, than men by the lack of funds for their medical education. Most who arrive at medical school are not from the lower economic classes (note the professions of their parents listed in Chapter 2), but even a girl from a relatively high-income background may be deterred from studying medicine by the knowledge that her financial backing will be cut short once she has received her bachelors degree. If it is a question of supporting a boy or girl through graduate studies, the money will nearly always go to the son. In addition, according to Dr. Edithe Levit, Assistant Director of the National Board of Medical Examiners, "The male student is more likely to be financed by his wife than the woman by her husband, unless he is much further along in his education." The situation of the husband established in a substantial wage-earning profession while his wife is still in medical school occurs with less and less frequency. Constance Smith, Dean of the Radcliffe Institute, reports that three-fourths of the women physicians who are receiving financial assistance for medical training through the Institute "are married to doctors at about the same level, so that where there is indebtedness, it is doubled."

[7] Marion E. Altenderfer and Margaret D. West, *How Medical Students Finance Their Education,* U.S. Department of Health, Education, and Welfare, Public Health Service publication no. 1336 (June, 1965), p. 30.

A survey of the expenses of medical students during 1963–64 showed male students to have higher expenses than female students—if single or married with no children. However, among those students who were married with one or more children and those who were divorced, widowed, or separated, women's expenses were higher than the men's. Table 5–3 below reproduces the breakdown of the expenses of women and men students during the 1963–64 academic year.

TABLE 5–3.   AVERAGE ANNUAL EXPENSES OF MEDICAL
STUDENTS BY MARITAL STATUS AND SEX

Marital status	Both sexes	Male	Female
Single	$2,713	2,722	2,617
Widowed, divorced, separated	3,581	3,498	3,804
Married, no children	4,797	4,813	4,360
Married, one child	4,876	4,870	5,223
Married, two or more children	5,244	5,226	6,334
total (average)	$3,577	$3,619	$3,003

Source: Marion E. Altenderfer and Margaret D. West, *How Medical Students Finance Their Education*, U.S. Department of Health, Education, and Welfare, Public Health Service publication no. 1336 (June, 1965), Table 15.

The authors state: "The higher expenses for female students with children reflects to some extent the necessity of employing baby-sitters or otherwise providing for child care while the mother is attending medical classes."[8] These expenses, often amounting to a full-time, semi-professional salary, are a thorn in the side of nearly all mothers in medicine—as well as in other professions—and may account partially for the higher attrition rate among mother-students. It has been suggested many times that household help be made tax-deductible for a working or studying woman, to facilitate her continuing in her profession.

The accumulation of large debts upon graduation can severely deter a "normal" family life for those couples who were not able to

[8] *Ibid.*, p. 16.

gain nonrefundable assistance during their medical school years. At the very time they should be paying back the loan money— three years after graduation, for the Health Professions Loans— they are at the age when they usually want to have their children. (The average medical student graduates at 26 or 27, completes his internship a year later, and then prepares to begin three-to-five years of residency at a salary ranging from $4,000 to $7,000 a year.) The prospect of an interminable delay in planning a family until all debts are paid has led some couples simply to have the children while in medical school—and come what may![9]

The general attitude of those in charge of student finances is that scholarships are to be given on the basis of need and competence only—without regard to sex, race, or creed. Dr. Lewis Thomas, Dean of New York University School of Medicine, reported that this was the case at his school, but added: "My impression is, however, that the women who come here are not in financial difficulties." According to Dean Thomas, most of his applicants came from private women's colleges in the East, and had the financial backing of their parents. A comparison of family background with debts for college and medical school education revealed that while 41 per cent of the students from families in the lowest income levels had debts upon graduation from medical school, only 5 per cent of the students from families in the highest quarter ($25,000 or more) had such debts.[10] Thus, it is probably true that single women students—generally supported by their families —do not, with their present background, require the same proportion of financial assistance as the men.

Some medical school administrators have stated that when a girl requires financial aid from outside sources in order to stay free from

[9] In the academic year 1963–64, out of 31,647 medical students, 59 per cent were single, 1 per cent divorced, and 40 per cent married. The 40 per cent who were married included 24 per cent with no children, 9 per cent with one child, and 7 per cent with two or more children. See Ceithaml, "The financial state of the American medical student," p. 498.

[10] Altenderfer and West, *How Medical Students Finance Their Education*, p. 69.

debt, they go out of their way to see that she gets it. They do not like the idea of a woman graduating with a "negative dowry," because it hinders her chance of finding a good marriage partner; a woman without debts will bring in more on the marriage market, they assume—probably correctly—than one with five-to-ten thousand dollars to be paid back by her and her husband's future earnings.

Debts upon graduation obviously have some ill affects on men, though in a different way than injuring their marital eligibility. Money-grabbing in the medical profession—a persistent public complaint—and jammed, long schedules, which make it impossible to give each patient adequate attention, are often seen as solutions by the young practitioner to the heavy debts in the years following graduation. By the time the physician is 35 or 40 years old, and finally free from debt, it is not likely that he will drastically cut his fees or overload. The habit of 80-hour "service" has already been formed.

The financing of medical education must be changed for both men and women. When a man with a lower-class background can see medical school as a feasible alternative, then women with equally small resources will be able to think of becoming physicians. In 1959, the United States Public Health Service predicted that a 30 per cent increase in physicians would be needed by 1975 in order to maintain the ratio of 149 doctors to 100,000 population; by 1963, the number of graduating physicians had increased only 7 per cent.[11] To solve the manpower shortage new groups of potential physicians will have to be tapped, and expanded financial aid opportunities for medical students will be necessary.

Women in Men's Schools

Most women medical students express reluctance to support any recruitment program which would increase significantly the proportion of women in their schools. The training is difficult, they

[11] "Manpower in the '60's." *Health Manpower Source Book* (Washington: U.S. Department of Health, Education, and Welfare, 1964), sec. 18.

say, demanding much emotional preparation. It is not a field for those who need to be coaxed into it or who might choose it on a whim. The stringent process of natural selection which occurs in the preceding years is necessary, they feel, to ensure that those girls who reach medical school are prepared to give what the training demands. In addition, many women openly admit that they enjoy their minority status. It accounts for the certain niceties extended to each girl and gives her a sense of being special—not just another faceless student lost in the crowd.

Dr. Helen Glaser reported at the Macy Conference on Women for Medicine that many girls in her questionnaire group felt that it was definitely an advantage to be a woman in medical school. "A predominant theme was that because of their sex they enjoyed more pleasant treatment by both fellow students and faculty than they felt was accorded the men students. They described their teachers and colleagues as 'more courteous, more polite, concerned, respectful, patient, encouraging, considerate, kinder, more gentle, easier and less abusive.'" Dr. Glaser added, "The opportunity for male-female interaction in a predominately male community was cited as a source of enjoyment, particularly where they felt they had maintained a clearly feminine role."

The women respondents in the Glasers' sample were not without complaints about their reception. Some felt that they were singled out by their instructors, that their errors were more easily noticed and remembered, and that every failure on their part was ascribed to their sex. Others thought that their work was not taken seriously by their instructors, that the faculty expectations of them were lower than for the men, and that a lower level of performance was accepted, thus stifling incentive to do well. On the other hand, a few felt that faculty expectations of them were higher than for the men, and that in fact they were required to work harder and to do better in order to be accepted as having done the same kind of job.

According to Dr. Glaser, respondents to the questionnaire revealed "an ambivalence about being thought of as one of the boys . . . and then consequently, as a result of that identification, being thought of as less of a woman. They expressed vague anxiety about being a member of the third sex." Some of this confusion may come from their minority position: medical school lecturers automatically address their audiences as "gentlemen" or "you guys," a phenomenon which is universally noted by women students. But most treat it as a joke, knowing that it is an understandable mistake and proud that they can accept it with humor.

Several women students who were interviewed observed that from the first day of medical school, the girls divided themselves between two groups: those who "act as if there is no minority problem," always sit with the boys, choose them as lab partners, and search for them in the cafeteria, and those who sit with other girls in classes, labs, and at meals, and are generally willing to identify with and draw comfort from those of their own sex. While the first offers a "buddy-buddy" casual relationship with the opposite sex, it can have drawbacks. One woman student remarked of her friend, "She acts as if she's one of the boys all day long and then wonders why none of them ever think of getting serious about her." Whatever the individual approach, women students find it necessary to make some adjustment in their relationships to male students. Some have an easier time excelling when they minimize sexual differences, while others appear to function better by creating a tiny girls' enclave within the larger student body.

For a minority of women who do not have outgoing personalities, the years of medical school can be extremely lonely ones, with few members of their sex as classmates and exclusion from total participation in the kinds of relaxation which unify male students. Even the most extroverted types will find themselves excluded at times. No matter how much a girl may want to prove that she is "one of the boys," sooner or later "dirty jokes" or rowdy demonstrations will present a situation from which she has to withdraw as a lady—and some men are not really at ease until they have verified that the line exists. The raucousness and cynicism in the dissection room, for which medical students have been notorious and which is quite understandable as a defense against their exposure to harsh physical realities, can repel a reserved girl, while others who are less prudish may feel utterly confused as to how far they are expected to participate. The woman medical student often finds herself in the position of pretending not to have seen some little piece of joking, or of acknowledging it with the faintest of smiles.

The problem of femininity looms large in an environment where one must excel and compete with male colleagues. Several Deans mentioned in interviews that they saw the crisis in female identity as one of the greatest problems of the woman medical student. The concessions a woman makes to retain this identity may take many forms. Dr. Jacqueline Parthemore, an intern at New York Hospital–Cornell University Medical Center, said at the Macy Conference:

> One thing that I learned as a woman in medical school was how to be tactful. The public high school graduate is, I think, taught a certain competitive spirit and a certain hands-up first with the right answer. I found that once you get to medical school this is no longer socially acceptable among the people with whom you're working. It isn't right for a woman to have her hand up first with the right answer. It is probably a sorry state of affairs to say that sometimes I kept my mouth shut when others of the girls in my class didn't. I am not sure that this is right. It may reflect social standards that are imposed on us and accepted while we are in med school.

One of the deterrents to excelling for many girls is the effect it will have on their social life. A second-year male medical student recently told me of an incident in his class which had irked him. One of the girls, an exceptional student, had been engaged to another medical student who stood much lower academically than she. Apparently the two had had difficulties over this discrepancy, or at least the girl had feared trouble, because on the last pathology exam she had tried to fail herself—succeeding only in getting a low grade—in order to block her chances of getting honors in the subject. "That's what I can't stand about women medical students!" the man who told the story exclaimed. "They're always lousing themselves up, holding back their intelligence so that no one will think they're competing."

Competition in the first two years of medical school is particularly troublesome, as it centers around an overwhelming number of facts which students must accumulate before each examination. A third-year student remarked on the tension she had experienced: "At first, everyone is so on edge that whoever is a little different bears the brunt, and the girls are definitely different and they have a hard time. Everything eases up by the second year, and even a little by the second semester of the first year. The boys know they won't be kicked out, and they grow to trust the girls a little."

In the clinical phase of medical school (usually the third and fourth years), new qualities are demanded, and the atmosphere of competition is lessened for most female medical students. To her male colleagues, the fact that a woman may have a way with patients is far less aggravating than would have been her *A* or Honors in the preceding two years. "Things have eased up quite a lot since we can't compete so directly any more," testified a fourth-year student. The disappearance of such rigorous competition may be one reason why medical school professors report that some of their women medical students suddenly seem to blossom and excel with the start of clinical contact.

*   *   *   *

Although every profession has its set of standards and values which its members learn to maintain, medicine, by its very nature, imposes on the students an even stricter sense of proprieties. From freshman year on, a large part of the medical student's training is to divine what the mores are and to adjust to them as quickly as possible. For instance:

> Suppose I should talk real enthusiastically about the job of dissection I did [a freshman explains]. Well, Earl will say, "Gee, I'm a great guy, too, you know," or something to that effect. From that remark I can tell I'm bragging too much. That cues me in, so I make a mental note not to brag so much the next time . . . Because you don't talk about your success to the group as a whole. It's sort of understood that you don't try to impress each other . . . A lot of the fellows belittle themselves . . . I mean, a fellow will say, for example, that he thought a certain structure was a

lymph node and that it turned out to be something entirely different. Then he and everyone else will laugh a lot over that . . .[12]

A woman student who was asked if she found medical school more difficult because of her sex replied, "You have to hold yourself in check a great deal.—But then so much of medicine *is* exactly this kind of self-control. We're all trained not to show our feelings, so it doesn't make that much difference whether you're a man or woman."

The comment of a third-year student illustrates this control, which becomes transferred from relationships with colleagues into patient contact, once clinical work begins:

> To say that a patient "searches your face" for clues is no overstatement. An example—while on OB, when trying to palpate a baby once, I got a little confused and frowned in puzzlement. I sensed at once that the mother saw the frown and was alarmed. So, I reassured her that everything was all right. I have always tried to remember not to do it again . . .[13]

"The process of learning to be a physician," states Robert Merton, "can be conceived as largely the learning of blending seeming or actual incompatibles into a consistent and stable pattern of professional behavior."[14] Merton gives an extensive list of these norms governing the physician's self-image, his relations to his patients, and his relations to colleagues and to the community. The following are only representative samples:

> The physician must maintain a self-critical attitude and be disciplined in the scientific appraisal of evidence. *But*: he must be decisive and not postpone decisions beyond what the situation requires, even when the scientific evidence is inadequate.
>
> The physician should have a strong moral character with abiding

[12] René Fox, "Training for uncertainty," in Robert Merton, J. Reader, and P. Kendall (eds.), *The Student Physician* (Cambridge: Harvard University Press, 1957), p. 220.

[13] *Ibid.*, p. 227.

[14] Robert K. Merton, "Some preliminaries to a sociology of medical education," in *The Student Physician*, p. 72.

commitments to basic moral values. *But*: he must avoid passing moral judgments on patients.

The physician must have a sense of autonomy; he must take the burden of responsibility and act as the situation, in his best judgment, requires. *But*: autonomy must not be allowed to become complacency or smug self-assurance; autonomy must be coupled with a due sense of humility.

The physician must be emotionally detached in his attitudes toward patients, keeping "his emotions on ice" and not becoming "overly identified" with patients. *But*: he must avoid becoming callous through excessive detachment, and should have compassionate concern for the patient.

The physician must respect the reputation of his colleagues, not holding them up to obloquy or ridicule before associates or patients. *But*: he is obligated to see to it that high standards of practice are maintained by others in the profession as well as by himself.[15]

Since intelligent women from childhood on become experienced at handling contradictory signals and goals—how to be intellectually productive while remaining feminine, for instance—they will be able in some cases to accomplish the needed balance with less strain than men. For the male student, who until now could turn his aggressive energy directly into individualistic intellectual endeavors, this sudden bridling of his personality may be difficult to bear. Student protests against the way medical schools are run come from male students, and rarely from women, who have long ago learned "passive acceptance" of their situation. David McClelland describes women as "field dependent" or "passive acceptant," and states that they are more likely to deal with the given context than men.[16]

[15] *Ibid.*, pp. 73–75.

[16] The rod-frame test is an example of an experiment conducted which bears out this fact (Witkin, 1954). In adjusting a rod inside a slightly tilted frame, women were more likely to use the frame as their relative reference (placing the rod in a position perpendicular to the frame), while men tended to use the ground alone, preferring a more absolute perpendicularity. See David McClelland, "Wanted: a new image for women," in Robert Lifton (ed.), *The Woman in America* (New York: Houghton Mifflin, 1964), p. 179.

Female students may also complain about medical school, but typically they add alongside their complaints that there must be a reason why the school maintains whatever irks them, or that things really aren't so bad on the whole. It would take a rare woman to initiate the drastic or even common-sense pragmatic proposals such as those made by male students throughout the country. The leaders of the second-year class at the University of Wisconsin Medical School, for instance, protested against the rapidity with which they were supposed to take class notes, which turned them into "shorthand machines" unable to listen to and think about the lectures. Several hours were then spent after class in which students compared their notes and tried to compile an accurate set. The class officers asked—along with other recommendations—that lecture notes be provided to alleviate this problem.

Eleanor Maccoby, a psychologist at Stanford University, suggests that the intellect of a woman is best suited for performing well-learned tasks, and that the anxiety of reconciling the conventions appropriate to her sex with those qualities needed for good analytic thinking (dominance, independence, active striving) usually has an adverse effect on her ability to think creatively or break new ground.[17] The anxiety experienced by every medical student as he or she learns to incorporate the conflicting values mentioned earlier results in a similar loss in creative thinking, which is actually suited to the rote learning of medical school. The difficulty arises within those students who were not prepared to subject themselves to such a complete hold on their personalities.

The actual process of studying may, in many cases, be easier for a woman than for a man. The diligent female student—who is accustomed from the beginning of college to spend her days in the laboratory and her evenings in the library—can often, by dogged work, maintain a good rank in her class. It is not genius that deter-

[17] This may account for the fact that many women prefer to practice medicine rather than to do research in the field. See Eleanor Maccoby, "Women's intellect," in Seymor M. Farber and Roger H. L. Wilson (eds.), *The Potential of Woman* (New York: McGraw-Hill [paperback], 1963), p. 37.

mines success during this period, and to the extent that work habits are more likely to have been formed in the female student, she may do very well without suffering a crisis of opposition to the workload. What was looked down on as being a "grind" in high school and college is now the most sensible way to get through.

A comparison of the scores of women and men medical students on the Edwards Personal Preference Schedule shows several differences in the two sexes, which may account for the ability of some women to get along in, or even to adjust smoothly to, the difficult medical school situation. As measured by the heterosexuality scale, women medical students are significantly lower than the men in their need for participation in activities with the opposite sex and are also nearly a standard deviation lower than their female colleagues in the general college group.[18] The lower "heterosexuality" score may be less an indication of the woman student's lack of desire for such contact, than of her capacity for sublimating as long as the situation is difficult. The hours of classes and work in the libraries leave little time for seeing men, especially those outside of medical school. Though one hears sarcastic comments occasionally that a major motive of women students in entering med school is to land a husband, it is impossible to believe that anyone would follow such an arduous path in order to achieve marital goals. Girls who want to meet eligible bachelor doctors would just as easily enter nursing and spare themselves the rigid preparation.

Woman's Medical College

For nearly seventy years, the Woman's Medical College of Pennsylvania has been the only medical school to educate women exclusively. Woman's Medical graduates three times as many women physicians as any other college or university, public or private, and nearly 8 per cent of the women doctors in the United States today have been educated at the College. Although a large proportion of the students have come from Pennsylvania, New York, New Jer-

---

[18] Hutchins, "Minorities, manpower, and medicine," p. 5.

sey and Massachusetts, nearly every state in the union has been represented, and Woman's Medical has educated foreign students as well.

The desire of most American women to receive their medical education alongside the men, however, has until quite recently hindered Woman's Medical College from attracting first-rate applicants. Except for a small minority of women who could have qualified for entrance in one of the coeducational medical colleges but preferred to attend Woman's Medical, this school has found itself often left with late deciders, older women, or women who felt they could not pass the entrance requirements of the other schools. In some ways, the College encouraged this second-class position by never having had the confidence to develop unique strengths of its own: it expended its energies trying to duplicate the predominately male schools on all fronts at once, under the assumption that any differences which existed between Woman's Medical and the coeducational medical schools could only show that the women were behind.

In the past several years, the image of Woman's Medical has begun to change rapidly. Upon assuming his post as Dean and President of the College in 1964, Dr. Glen Leymaster felt that he had to make one of two choices: either to turn the College into a coeducational school, or to justify it on its own terms. Dr. Leymaster chose the latter. In describing the premise behind the changes he hopes to institute, Leymaster states: "While there can be no compromise with quality, there can be variation among medical schools in relative emphasis among disciplines. All branches of medicine must be open to individual students, but a medical school with a unique student body ought to have unusual strength in some areas and thus provide unusual opportunities for its students."[19]

As a first step in this policy, the Departments of Pediatrics,

[19] Glen R. Leymaster, "An answer: a national center for medical education for women—forecast or fantasy?" *J. Amer. Med. Wom. Ass.* 20, no. 4 (1965):347.

Psychiatry, and Physiology have been strengthened, with the ulti-
mate goal of attracting first-rate women who are interested in these
particularly "feminine" fields. The specialties of psychiatry and
pediatrics have together attracted nearly 35 per cent of the women
receiving Board certification,[20] and it is appropriate that Woman's
Medical should establish itself strongly in these fields.

In seeking to deal with the special problems of women students,
Woman's Medical has established a policy of flexibility: time-off is
given for pregnancy, and if a woman knows she will have to
leave school for the months when a particular subject is offered,
she is allowed to take it beforehand or after. The object is always
to help her as far as possible to blend her needs as a wife and
mother with her career in medicine.

As an integral part of the College, Woman's Medical is also in
the process of establishing a National Retraining Center for those
women who have been forced to take time off during the years of
child-rearing and who need a period of reacquaintance with the
field before continuing their education or reentering a responsible
professional position. Several women have already gone through
retraining there as part of a pilot program, rapidly covering the
material alongside their younger colleagues. One woman, who had
dropped out after her internship to raise two children, returned to
the Department of Physiology for the first several months, where
she taught the subject to nurses while reacquainting herself with
the terminology and practice of medicine. The presence of these
women on campus gives the younger students an often much-
needed model.

This new program is in keeping with Dr. Leymaster's intention
to turn the college into an experimental center:

> The nation needs an institution primarily, not incidentally, con-
> cerned with attracting women into medicine, with attempting to
> solve the educational problems of the woman medical student,
> and with the continuing education of the woman physician. These
> are problems for all schools, but one institution can perform an

[20] Hutchins, "Minorities, manpower, and medicine," Table 8.

important service as a pace setter by identifying the problems, by innovating, and by experimenting with a variety of solutions."[21]

How does the student body feel about attending a school where there are only women students? (In the strict sense, there are some men: since 1953, several male students have been accepted each year into graduate programs in the medical sciences.) Random talks with students at the College revealed that the women are excited about the changes being made and would generally be against their school becoming coeducational. A freshman, one of the new type of student the College has started to attract, commented on the *esprit de corps* which she felt in her class. A senior remarked that she was happy that there was "one school which genuinely cares about women getting a medical education." Another student testified, "I'm glad to be in a school where I don't have to compete with men." Her closest friend, she said, was at Jefferson Medical College, and at times found it a strain to balance the friendly in-school relationships with men and the more serious ones on the outside. "I feel that I have the run of all the medical schools in the Philadelphia area," said the girl, "and I don't have to worry about carrying my social life into the classroom."

Woman's Medical College's main problem is financial. Not being part of a university or state educational system, it is confronted with the same endowment struggle which affects most private colleges. In addition, women are not always the most generous alumni, often deferring to their husbands' decision of which college to support. Recent foundation grants have helped the College with some of its new programs, including greatly expanded clinical and hospital facilities. As several studies have shown, there is a positive correlation between the level of finance of a school and the ability and success of a student body,[22] and it is particularly important that Woman's Medical receives increased support of this type.

[21] Leymaster, "An answer: a national center for medical education for women—forecast or fantasy?" p. 347.

[22] Johnson and Hutchins, "Doctor or dropout? A study of medical student attrition," *J. Med. Educ.* 41, no. 12 (1966):1159.

VI

THE MEDICAL SCHOOL DROPOUT

In nearly all programs beyond the college level, women have had a higher rate of attrition than men, a fact which has been the source of ambivalence and hesitation among deans and admissions officers as well as foundations awarding grants for higher education. The higher attrition rate has been particularly serious among women in graduate programs.

> At Columbia University, for example, only about 2 to 3 per cent of the women who became doctoral candidates in 1945–51 had earned the doctor's degree by 1956, as compared with 5 to 13 per cent of the men who had. At Radcliffe College, the annual attrition rate for women at all stages of graduate study was 17 per cent in 1959–60; only one student out of every ten enrolled received the doctorate. Even among Woodrow Wilson fellows, highly selected as they were, the attrition rate for women in 1958–59 was twice that for men.[1]

There are two differences between the attrition patterns of women medical students and women in other graduate studies. In the first place, women medical school students, although they have had nearly twice as high an attrition rate as male medical students, still have one of the lowest rates of attrition among women seeking higher degrees. About 85 per cent of all of the women who enter medical school receive their M.D. degrees. (Medicine itself has a dropout rate of only 9 per cent of its students, in comparison with 40 per cent of all law school entrants, 50 per cent of all engineering

[1] Jessie Bernard, *Academic Women* (Cleveland: Meridian, 1966), pp. 58–59.

students, an estimated 15-to-20 per cent of all theology students, and 44 per cent of nursing school degree candidiates.)[2]

The second difference is that of the women who drop out of medical school, more than two-thirds do so in the first year. Apparently once this period is completed, academic difficulties become negligible and personal complications have a smaller effect.

Among women medical students, the most important causes of attrition are "nonacademic."[3] Of the women, 8 per cent—compared with only 3 per cent of the men—reported that they were in good academic standing when they left medical school. On the other hand, the difference in percentage of academic dropouts among both sexes is not so great: while attrition due to academic difficulties accounts for 5 per cent of the male students, it makes

TABLE 6–1. ATTRITION BY SEX, 1949–58 ENTRANTS

Sex	Total entrants		Academic dropouts		Nonacademic dropouts		Total dropouts	
	no.	(per cent)	no.	(per cent)	no.	(per cent)	no.	(per cent)
Male	71,140	94.28	3,541	4.98	2,346	3.30	5,887	8.28
Female	4,313	5.72	316	7.33	353	8.18	669	15.51
Total	75,453	100.00	3,867	5.11	2,699	3.58	6,556	8.69

Source: Davis G. Johnson and Edwin B. Hutchins, "Doctor or dropout? A study of medical student attrition," *J. Med. Ed.* 41, no. 12 (1966):1140.

[2] Davis G. Johnson and Edwin B. Hutchins, "Doctor or dropout? A study of medical student attrition." *J. Med. Educ.* 41, no. 12 (1966): 1116.

[3] Although the terms "academic" and "nonacademic" dropouts imply a differentiation which need not exist—one student who disliked medical school might simply stop studying, while another would take himself out before receiving a notice of failure—for the purposes of analyses in this chapter, the AAMC definitions will be used: an "academic" dropout will mean "any student who was in academic difficulty at the time he was dismissed or withdrew from medical school"; a "nonacademic" dropout will denote "any student who was not in academic difficulty at the time he left." See *ibid.*, p. 1132.

up only slightly more than 7 per cent of the female students. Table 6–1 gives a breakdown of attrition by sex for all 1949–58 entrants of United States medical schools.

Thus, women proved to be about as good students as men, the statistical difference being almost negligible. The greater risk they posed as medical candidates was in the nonacademic area.

The reasons for the greater attrition among women students are most commonly said to be marriage and pregnancy. Interestingly enough, unpublished data from an AAMC study by Johnson and Hutchins[4] of medical school dropouts showed that this was not the case. Of the nonacademic dropout group 67 per cent were single, and 81 per cent had no children. Of those who did have children, only 31 per cent of the nonacademic group stated that having children had been a factor in causing them to drop out.

Being married by itself appears to have no harmful—indeed, perhaps even a beneficial—effect on a woman's progress in medical school. According to the AAMC data, there was relatively little difference in the marital status of those who made regular progress and those who did not. In fact, the highest proportion of married women was found in the regular student group (32 per cent). Among those women who were forced to repeat a year or more for academic reasons, 8 per cent were married. Twenty-seven per cent of the academic dropouts and 28 per cent of the nonacademic dropouts were also married women, which is a higher proportion than among the repeaters but less than among the group which made regular progress. The point of marriage in the woman's education —before or during medical school—seems to have had no relationship to her scholastic progress.

---

[4] The data in this chapter on women dropouts come from 187 replies of 1961–62 women medical students, including 10 per cent of the regular students of all U.S. medical schools (122) and all the irregular students (12 repeaters, 22 academic, and 31 nonacademic dropouts), to selected items on the 12-page AAMC Attrition Study questionnaire. A special list of women students was made by the Association of American Medical Colleges at the author's request.

The presence of children, however, does show up as a significant factor in the nonacademic dropout group: 19 per cent of the non-academic dropouts reported having one or more children, in contrast to 9.2 per cent of the regular students, 8.3 per cent of the repeaters, and only 4.5 per cent of the academic dropouts. (Virtually all of the mother-students in all groups had no more than one child.) Considering that the two lowest rates of having children were among repeaters and academic dropouts, it would appear that academic difficulties have other causes. It is true that nonacademic dropouts had the highest frequency of children, but the second highest group was the regulars. Although children may present a conflict of duties which the hitherto successful woman student believes can only be resolved through a temporary abandonment of her career, there are additional factors which make children a crucial obstacle for some and a minor setback for others.

For most medical students, the decision to have a child can be made quite rationally, taking into consideration other aspects of the couple's position in life. Surveys of medical students have shown that they are, in many cases, as naïve as the general public on matters of family planning. However, only 10 per cent of the female nonacademic dropouts reported that they had left school because of marriage or pregnancy. Interviews with women medical students corroborate this data, and indicate that there is a good deal of planning on the woman's side. In fact, after deciding that a child was wanted, most women scheduled their pregnancies carefully so that little time would be taken out from their studies.

It may be that with the actual appearance of the child whose so obvious needs make a strong appeal to full maternal attention, some women who had actually planned to continue their training begin to consider dropping out. On the other hand—to propose a less generous explanation—it could be that a woman predicts the extent to which she will feel herself drawn to devote herself to her child, and thus sees its birth as a means of easing out of the professional world. In other words, nonacademic dropouts may have a higher rate of children because they, as a group, were reluctant all along to become high-geared professional women.

The role model provided by the woman medical student's mother appears to be important in her own ability to cope with her studies in addition to having children, as Table 6–2 indicates. As might be predicted, the academic and nonacademic dropouts had the highest proportion of housewife mothers, while the regular students and repeaters had a substantial percentage of mothers in professional, semi-professional, and managerial fields. Having had a working mother gives the young woman a model for combining a career with marriage and eventually, children. On the other hand, those students with housewife-mothers may suddenly experience a strong, mysterious pull to raise a family and take care of the house when they become twenty-two, which they may not have anticipated as bright, ambitious, nineteen-year-old pre-meds. It is almost as if they wake up in anatomy lab and sense that something is wrong— they are not repeating their mother's pattern.

TABLE 6–2. OCCUPATION OF MOTHER: 1961–62 WOMEN STUDENTS

	Regular	Repeater	Academic dropout	Non-academic dropout
	N–122	N–12	N–22	N–31
	(per cent)	(per cent)	(per cent)	(per cent)
Professional, semi-professional managerial (except M. D.)	24	42	18	3.2
Physician	2.5	—	—	—
Other medical	1.6	8.3	—	3.2
Proprietor	1.6	—	—	—
Clerical and sales	10.6	8.3	9	12.9
Service	1.6	—	—	3.2
Agriculture, fishing, forestry	—	—	—	—
Skilled	1.6	8.3	—	9.0
Semi-skilled	1.6	—	—	3.2
Unskilled	2.3	—	—	—
Housewife	50.0	33.3	73.0	64.5

The disproportionately high percentage of working mothers and physician relatives among the repeater group is notable. (Fifty-nine per cent had one or more physician relatives, in contrast to 41 per cent of the regular students, 36 per cent of the academic dropouts,

and 29 per cent of the nonacademic dropouts.) It suggests that
many of the repeaters might have been academic dropouts had
they not had working mothers and physicians among their relatives. Conversely, some of the academic and nonacademic dropouts
might have been saved if they had come from environments which
more actively fostered their career.

Various background factors were found in the AAMC study to
be associated with either regular progress or attrition. The successful students more commonly came from urban backgrounds and
went to colleges which had extensive pre-medical programs. They
had higher MCAT scores and a larger proportion had been pre-
medical or science majors.[5] Among the intellectual characteristics
of medical students, the women came out fairly well-prepared and
capable.

However, some of the nonintellectual characteristics related to
higher attrition potential in the AAMC study showed up more
frequently among women medical students than among men. In a
comparison of women and men first-year medical students on the
same test, women showed less need for achievement, dominance,
and aggression, and more of a deference need[6]—characteristics
which were also associated with attrition. Scores on the Edwards
Personal Preference Schedule established academic dropouts as
"significantly less achievement-oriented. Perhaps in an effort to
compensate for this, they tend also to be more deferent and less
aggressive and to exact a higher degree of orderliness."[7] On the
dominance scale, "regular students on the average exhibited a
higher need for dominance than did their colleagues who withdrew from medical school in good academic standing."[8]

Because the traits associated with attrition are traditionally fem-

[5] Johnson and Hutchins, "Doctor or dropout?" pp. 1145–49.
[6] Edwin B. Hutchins, "Minorities, manpower, and medicine," Division
of Education, Association of American Medical Colleges, Technical Report no. S–663 (1966), Table 6.
[7] Johnson and Hutchins, "Doctor or dropout?" p. 1151.
[8] *Ibid.*

inine, women stand a greater chance of dropping out than men—irrespective of the difficulty of absorbing the curriculum or of combining marriage and medicine. Aggression and dominance (often associated with intellectual performance)[9] are frowned upon in women, and the need to achieve has simply not been developed to as great an extent in women as in men. In addition, since women can receive achievement gratification for having and raising children, this may occasionally dissipate the need for achievement in intellectual areas.

*   *   *   *

The predictive value of these factors may interest admissions officers, who understandably look for guides to a better selection of medical school candidates, but it is certainly not the aim of this chapter to set up more obstacles to women entering medicine than already exist. It would be a step in the wrong direction to encourage the selection of only those girls whose fathers are physicians, who scored high on dominance tests, who come from urban areas, or whose mothers worked at some point in their lives. The emphasis on creating more and more refined tools for selection may, in any case, be too narrow an approach to the dropout problem.

In this respect, it should be noted that the combined rate of attrition among all students has been rising "from a low of less than 7 per cent for those admitted in 1950 to an estimated high of nearly 11 per cent for those who entered in 1961."[10] This increase has been distributed equally among women and men students, and has to do with a combination of factors—both inside and outside medical schools. While, as Johnson and Hutchins state, "attrition per se should not necessarily be completely eliminated,"[11] a rising dropout rate is cause for alarm and extremely wasteful in the face of the public's expanded need for medical services. With the pro-

[9] Eleanor Maccoby, "Women's intellect," in Seymor M. Farber and Roger H. L. Wilson (eds.), *The Potential of Woman* (New York: McGraw-Hill, 1963).

[10] Johnson and Hutchins, "Doctor or dropout?" p. 1117.

[11] *Ibid.*, p. 1115.

jected increase in the number of medical students to be trained in the next years, it is particularly important to focus on the potential sources of medical school attrition.

Early studies of this problem tended to accentuate inferior pre-medical preparation, personal background, and other factors having to do with limitations of the *students*. It is only in the last decade, and particularly with the Johnson and Hutchins study, that the medical school environment itself has come under scrutiny as a possible explanation of attrition. Since "trend data from the MCAT program indicate that measured ability has remained stable or in-creased over the same period that attrition has increased,"[12] there is no reason to assume that medical schools are getting an intellec-tually inferior student. The differences seem to be in his or her emotional adjustment to medical school.

Within the medical school environment itself, attrition is prob-ably a twofold problem, resulting from an interaction between weaknesses in the student and the shortcomings of his school. Some schools have a persistently higher rate of attrition among their students than do others; and, while certain schools have more dropouts due to academic reasons, others have a higher proportion of nonacademic dropouts. In the AAMC sample of medical institu-tions, there were obvious attributes which characterized the high-attrition schools: their total operating budgets were often smaller, influencing the mean academic level of the student body; they were more likely to have restrictions on out-of-state students and less likely to have substantial funds for research; finally, the dis-crepancy between what administrators and students felt to be the source of attrition appeared to be the greatest in those schools with a high dropout rate, indicating a lack of communication between students and administration in these schools. In general, adminis-trators commonly felt that dropouts could be lessened through student-related factors such as pre-medical background, greater se-lectivity of students, and higher student morale. Changes in the schools themselves were not generally judged to be necessary.

[12] *Ibid.*, p. 1125.

The AAMC total student sample proved a great deal more critical of such features as curriculum, instruction, faculty-student relationships, student morale, and also, though to a lesser extent, student services (counseling, financial aid, housing, etc.). Interestingly, the women who answered the questionnaire were more inclined to agree with the deans that irregular progress had more to do with the students' problems than the school's inadequacies. Except for the repeater group, women students were less critical than men of curriculum and instruction. What they did emphasize —particularly nonacademic women dropouts—were: (1) being bothered by academic and psychological pressures of medical school; (2) emotional problems; (3) loneliness and unhappiness; (4) social and dating problems; (5) lack of time and effort on studies; (6) poor study habits; and (7) lack of confidence in ability to become a doctor. In answering a question about specific personal difficulties interfering with medical school progress, the irregular women students cited most of all their relationships with and dependence on parents, health problems, insecurities regarding the future, and relationships with the opposite sex.

All this is a far cry from the woman who drops out simply because of her dual role of homemaker and professional. While such a conflict may become increasingly important at later stages in the career of an aspiring woman physician, it cannot be said to be a crucial factor during medical school. Instead, a sensitivity which is perhaps more marked in women students to the tensions of the environment may affect their ability to make regular progress. This is borne out by the fact that women respondents to the AAMC questionnaire consistently rated counseling as an important area for the prevention of irregular progress—repeaters and academic dropouts assigned better counseling services 3.3 out of 4 in importance. Both men and women students rated counseling 2.76 in importance for the prevention of irregular progress, in contrast to the deans, who assigned it only 1.8.[13]

Given the particular difficulties which women face in medical

[13] *Ibid.*, pp. 1136, 1249.

school, it is especially important to offer effective counseling during these years. In a discussion on the subject at the Macy Conference on Women in Medicine, Dr. Joseph Gardella, Associate Dean of Harvard Medical School, stated:

> It is quite apparent, at least to me, that sometimes these emotional problems in women relate more to external factors than to internal ones. For this reason, I think, they are more or less easily managed. I think that part of their emotional problems is their identity as individuals in a largely male society, the fact that they have fewer models, strong models, whom they can emulate. Also, there are fewer people on the faculty with whom they can speak. I think very careful counseling through medical school is very important for women, perhaps a little bit more than for men, in view of their added problems.

Counseling in medical school, for either men or women, has usually been a very casual affair. The students are "free" to go to a faculty member or to the dean if they feel the need of someone to talk to. But since medical students are taught to show *equanimitas* at all times as the prime virtue of the physician, they may be reluctant to declare openly to their superiors their emotional difficulties if they have them, or to ask for more than the most perfunctory advice. It is hard to believe the claim of one dean that, "A lot of students come right to me with their problems." A student at his school testified, in fact, that all attempts to make appointments with him were referred to his assistant. In the case of women, their position of being "on trial" by a segment of faculty, administration, and students who are watching to see if they will deserve the places usurped from men would make it extremely unlikely for them to turn to these same watchdogs. And when they take the chance, they do not always find an impartial or sympathetic audience.

In their dropout study, Hutchins and Johnson cite the case of a female medical student who witnessed continual bickering and competition among the faculty for students' homework time, and finally felt that she could not remain in the tense situation:

> Morale was low, and we had tremendous losses that year. I know of one instance where there was a conscious effort on the part of

the faculty to retain a student, but this was an unusual case. I took a professor at his word and went to see him and came out more frustrated than I went in. He was most unhelpful. I think that schools need more people who take a personal interest in the students. I don't think much interest is taken in the student here, unless he goes to the Psychiatry Office. Members of the faculty are fairly approachable but show no genuine interest, and the Dean is much too busy with other things. He shouldn't have been though, because twelve of us were caught up in a conflict between two instructors. Nobody would believe this, but the real problem wasn't the inability of the students as much as the immaturity of the faculty.[14]

There has been a growing concern—along with the general upsurge of importance given to counseling—that these students have a highly-trained individual other than the staff psychiatrist to whom they can take their difficulties. (The hesitation to visit a psychiatrist is not only because of the potential stigma involved, but also because of the long-term orientation of psychotherapy.) Many educators have come to see the importance of providing the female students with a counselor of their own sex; being a minority group, women have special problems of adaptation in addition to practical difficulties such as housing (particularly in cities where schools are in high-crime-rate neighborhoods). A sensitive woman counselor, probably trained as a physician, could offer a model and help greatly with specific advice as well as give emotional support. While it has been suggested in earlier chapters that counseling is no panacea, it may be able to perform with substantially more effectiveness in the medical school environment, where the problem is to help generally superior students adapt to a situation whose difficulties are manifest and well-defined.

[14] *Ibid.*, p. 1111.

VII

THE WOMAN INTERN

From the standpoint of physical strain, the internship is the most difficult year for any man or woman training to become a physician. Because the program is extremely strenuous and usually inflexible in its structure, the period can place a heavy toll on a married woman and those dependent on her. Most women do complete, or at least begin, their internships, however, since in nearly all states the year of hospital training is required for licensure.

Although no data have been gathered comparing the stress of the internship on women and men, medical educators are firm in their belief that, especially if unmarried, a woman can perform her duties as well and as devotedly as a man. Evidence from other stressful situations suggests that women may actually have greater reserves than men. In London, during the World War II blitz, the incidence of emotional shock and psychoneuroses was 70 per cent higher in men than in women, while concentration camp reports indicate that women had fewer nervous breakdowns.[1] The comparison with stress in bombing and concentration camp situations is not as far-fetched as it may seem. A woman who had completed her internship at a large metropolitan hospital remarked, "It's like being on a battlefield. You're constantly bombarded by critical moments." The closely-quartered live-in situation, with little opportunity to stray outside the hospital, adds to the strain for both women and men.

In 1917 when Connie Guion, Bellevue's first woman doctor, took

[1] Morton Hunt, *Her Infinite Variety* (New York: Harper and Row, 1962), p. 33.

her internship, interns were required to ride behind the ambulances for 24 hours at a stretch. After a month or so of hanging on like this, Dr. Guion felt herself becoming physically rundown. Taking the initiative, she requested of the directors of the hospital that they decrease the number of hours demanded at one time. Soon after, realizing the justice of this human appeal, Bellevue cut the ambulance duty of interns to 12 hours. Today, the work requirements of interns vary widely from hospital to hospital. A prominent university-affiliated hospital, for instance, demands a schedule of 36 hours on duty and 12 off—still a strenuous schedule —with every other weekend free, while a nonaffiliated hospital which has greater difficulty filling its house staff positions may attract interns with more lenient conditions: one out of three or four nights on duty, and one weekend a month. Terraced apartments and baby-sitting provisions may be added to increase the bargaining power of an unaffiliated hospital, and some of these institutions have pioneered in special programs for mother-interns. However, the possibility of receiving better training at a teaching hospital, and the prestige attached to having attended an affiliated institution, sway most ambitious students in favor of longer hours and less pay.

An unmarried woman student, who had served a highly demanding clerkship which forced her to live in the hospital and spend alternate nights on duty, was considering a small unaffiliated hospital for her internship because of "the chance to live a somewhat more independent and normal life." This included, for her, being able to maintain her interest in music—going to concerts and practicing her violin. When she told her chief of service, he replied, "You really should go to a teaching hospital, just to prove that you deserve a good residency. It's only a year out of your life. . . . But then you're a girl," he added, "so maybe the strain would be too much . . ." Despite this bait, the woman decided to accept the position in the small hospital. She felt that the program was adequate for the residency she desired, and she was glad to get into a less strenuous situation.

Many women, whether because of higher aspirations or their fear of differentiating themselves from their male colleagues, would be reluctant to follow the woman described above. In fact, student physicians in general are not inclined to experiment with programs offered outside the stiffly structured ones of the affiliated hospitals. The Millis Report on Graduate Medical Education, which maintained that the internship no longer fulfills any educative use and should be abandoned, documented the attitude of American graduates in favor of the status quo: "In a study conducted by the Bureau of Applied Social Research of Columbia University, only a small minority of interns and residents felt they were being exploited, yet only about a quarter of them considered what they were learning to be very much worth the time spent providing services for the hospital."[2] Women residents who were questioned by me about their opinions regarding the internship admitted that it had been a period of hardship, but most reacted hesitantly toward any revisions suggested. Some tended to resent it when the subject of their having had difficulties was even broached.

Part of the reason for this attitude is the aura attached to the internship itself. Like a puberty rite through which all boys must pass in order to achieve their manhood, medical students look forward with pride and fear to the internship. (This applies equally to women medical students.) Where a rebellion on their part might have instigated changes in policy, they have supported the internship with little more opposition than the occasional complaining done by any soldier proud of and exhausted by the huge task he has taken on.[3]

If the intern intends to enter a residency in one of the more competitive specialties, such as internal medicine or surgery, an addi-

[2] The report of the Citizen's Commission on Graduate Medical Education, *The Graduate Education of Physicians* (American Medical Association, 1966), p. 59.

[3] In Japan and England—by contrast—interns have gone on strike several times in recent years against such conditions as the lack of financial stipends, poorly structured teaching programs, and the lack of opportunity to assume responsibility in patient care.

tional incentive for competing within the established system is provided, and he or she may go to extreme lengths to catch the eye and approval of his chief of service. A graduate of twenty years related with pleasure how, in order to impress the surgical department head where he hoped to take his residency, he had once spent 18 days straight without leaving the hospital, going several times for 72 hours at a stretch without sleep. "If I'd have cracked up, it would have been nobody's fault but mine," he laughed, "but at the time I thought it was great!"

Even the intern who aspires to an easily-gained residency position becomes caught up in the intensity of the hospital experience. The operating ethic for everyone is duty; a great deal of time is spent on-call in the hospital, in case an emergency should arise. To the question, "What do you do with your time off?" many interns simply reply, "Sleep."

Off-duty hours when awake are also spent in the hospital, joking with the staff, playing cards or snacking. The last is a particular hazard for women interns. An attractive single girl who was putting on too many pounds during her internship lamented that, "When you're up so much, there's just time for too many meals." Despite the fact that the internship involves hard work, there is little exercise to be gotten walking down hospital corridors, and the lack of fresh air and poor or irregular diet often gives the intern that puffy grayish look which is so commonly seen atop the white jackets in hospital elevators. A twenty-five-year-old woman intern, who was determined to preserve what she could of her youth, said that she spent her hours off, when she had enough energy to leave the hospital, roaming through cosmetic departments of the city's department stores and experimenting with facial creams and lotions.

The paralysis which keeps so many physicians in the hospital when they are free to leave is probably one of the most serious side-effects of the hospital-centered life. In the wards everyone knows the intern and understands his exhaustion, and there are relatively few demands of the type which require an expenditure of the involvement and emotion such as are often found on the outside.

A physician who had married another student during medical school and was divorced at the beginning of her residency, spoke rather frankly of the dissolution of her marriage. She explained:

> You're continually worn out. I always used to joke that my husband and I met in the elevator, in the lunch room, and in bed—occasionally. You let problems between you slide . . . You go out less—which you don't think matters at the time. People on the outside thought we were always driving ourselves so hard; but you'd be surprised, sometimes you even stay late because when you're really exhausted, it's much easier to hang around and chat with your buddies than to have to work with whatever's waiting at home. A lot of nights you waste time until you think your mate will be asleep so you can just crawl into bed beside the zonked-out body next to you. Have you ever seen a person stop off at every floor on the way down to say goodbye to everyone? It can take an awfully long time.

Although many marriages survive this difficult period, the threat imposed by the completeness of the internship experience is often great. Among men, the feeling of comradeship becomes strong, like being in the army, and often competes with their marital ties; wives of interns are notoriously discontented. Yearning to become part of the group, some women interns go to great lengths to be accepted at the pool table or in the lounge when the men are chatting. On the other hand, female interns, if they wish, find it much easier to separate themselves from the hospital once their work is over. Their exclusion from this buddy-buddy system has the advantage that it leaves them freer to pursue their personal lives. A common reaction is to feel relieved at the isolation, which is so rare in a dormitory situation. One woman who was asked about her cafeteria companions said, "I eat my lunch in the locker room, alone, and love it!" Mother-interns often use their free time to run home to be with their children. A woman who lived too far away to do this had her husband bring the children to see her for an hour on the nights she had to stay at the hospital.

The work itself—making rounds, running laboratory tests, working up histories—provides another set of problems for the female intern, some of them contingent on her marital state. For the single girl probably the most important balance she has to maintain is that of retaining her feminity while demonstrating her capacity for hard work. Unmarried women are more conscious of having to hold themselves back and to put their feminine charm to work than are the married women. "You should be good, but not too good," said an unmarried intern. Another, sensing the threat that she posed to the men in her unit, had adopted a manner of "I'm just in it for kicks," which the head of her department had actually come to believe. Stories are told in every hospital of women who play "Baby Face" in order to appear less competitive. Unfortunately, these masks collapse after long days with little or no sleep, and the women sometimes get themselves into trouble with their male colleagues as a result. "When you're tired, you can't play anything," said an older woman who had watched much of this type of behavior. "And the men don't like it when the sweet little girl becomes a pushy bitch at the end of a 36-hour stretch."

Josephine Williams, in her dissertation, "The Professional Status of the Woman Physician," summarizes the traditional model for relationships between male and female physicians: "With a male colleague, she should play the faithful assistant role, typified by the nursing ideal; she must be sensitive to his definition of the situation, and flexible in being feminine and businesslike by turns."[4] As with the successful women in many top-level professions, women in medicine often use "personal charm, subtle manipulation, fake naïvité, and other techniques which an admirer might call 'the human touch' and a detractor might call deceit."[5]

One afternoon while I was waiting to interview a young woman in the house staff lounge, a male doctor who was having his lunch there at the time began to talk with me. When he discovered the nature of my project, he heatedly attacked the whole idea of women entering medicine, saying that their place was in the home

[4] Josephine J. Williams, "The professional status of women in medicine" (unpublished Ph.D. dissertation, Department of Sociology, University of Chicago, 1949).

[5] Hunt, *Her Infinite Variety*, p. 260.

or in other professions. With one exception, he said, he had never known a woman doctor who was worthy of taking a man's position in any medical training program. He named the woman, and I was pleased to find that I had an appointment with her the next day. She was a pretty, petite young woman, who had married a non-professional. I spoke to her of the compliment she had received, and found she was not at all surprised by it. "Being on the ward is like being in a marriage," she observed. "If you're feminine and let them think *they're* making the decisions, you'll get along very well. Men don't like aggressive, crusading women." There had been only one time, she told me, when this particular doctor had been hostile towards her, and that was the previous year when she had been pregnant; but she had been able to show him, even then, that she could be depended on to do her share of the work.

Because the work is so obviously strenuous and the situation competitive, over-taxed male colleagues are often on the lookout for any admission of feminine weaknesses: menstrual cramps which might have slowed down the woman, a baby-sitter whose lateness forced her to postpone her own arrival at the hospital, or, most conspicuous, the swelling of the late months of pregnancy.

In the face of this mistrust, however, women interns claim they keep a grim muteness about their daily difficulties. "I would try as hard as possible not to say why I couldn't be on time," reported the mother of two young children, who had occasionally been forced to wait for her baby-sitter or, if the sitter didn't arrive, to drop a child off at a friend's house before coming to work. She noted that the men in her program could call in to say they'd be late because their car needed repairs, or could take an hour off during the day to run to the bank, and nobody would think anything of it. A common feeling among the mothers was that while the men could talk freely about their families during working hours, it was a good policy for a woman to keep her home life to herself and her baby pictures tucked in her pocket. Not doing so would prompt the accusation that she was a chatty mother who would be better off with the other women at home.

Some men who think women have an easier time of it complain

not of their work output, but of the amenities accorded to them.
Josephine Williams writes, "The most generally accepted criticism
[among men] is that 'women tend to demand equal rights without
assuming equal responsibility.' However, data . . . show that men
tend to exaggerate the special privileges that women claim"[6] The
men in her study checked more items on her list of "obligations of
a man to a woman" than did the women she sampled. Avoiding
dirty jokes, holding doors open, letting the woman examine the
patients first, and doing the messy clean-up work for her, were
among the privileges which men felt they were asked to extend,
but which the women thought they did not demand. It is highly
possible, of course, that some women come to expect feminine
privileges such as they have always received without being aware
of it, just as it is likely that the men offer these courtesies in order
to maintain their superiority. Most women, when asked by me
about whether the men in their programs extended such assistance,
tended to raise their eyebrows incredulously.

In her dissertation, Williams points out the contradictions of a
minority position: at the same time that equal rights are demanded,
unconscious tests are often made by the minority group in order to
reaffirm once again their own second-class status. She tells the
following story, which she had witnessed, as an example: A woman
student was complaining that a certain instructor deliberately
baited women students. When a male classmate challenged her,
she reminded him of the instructor's attempt to embarrass her that
morning in class. The man immediately asked her if she hadn't
been late to class, and she had to admit that she had.[7]

The other side of the same problem was told to me at an AMWA
party by a young woman intern. She had a male colleague who
worked fairly hard when he was on the job, but who never managed to arrive on time. One morning, after he had come in half an
hour late, the two of them were taking assignments, and he said:
"Marlene, are you *sure* you do your share?" Another female intern,

[6] Williams, "The professional status of women in medicine."
[7] *Ibid.*

standing nearby when the story was told, interjected at this point, "Well, *do* we?"—whereupon everyone at the party burst out laughing.

A perfect *reductio ad absurdum* of the equal rights versus equal privileges syndrome was reached in a 1935 Federal Civil Service order, which was reported by the Washington *Daily News*:

> Maternity leave was approved almost unanimously by the committee which drafted the regulations. The only opposition came from the women. Firm believers in equal rights, they contended that allowing maternity leave was discrimination in favor of women, which they believe is just as unpleasant as discrimination against women. A compromise was finally reached whereby no mention is made of sex in the maternity leave regulation.[8]

The difficulty of coming to the end of this vicious circle is probably one reason why women in medicine (as do many minority groups) try to ignore their minority status and disclaim any generalizations made of them. Although one young woman doctor commented when asked about it: "Denying the differences due to sex is like denying that a patient of yours is going to die," most of the women of the younger generation respond initially to questions in this area, as if the problems between the sexes were inconsequential. Almost all maintain that they can prove their worth and function rather unself-consciously within the department; they think that those few men who continue not to accept them must have their own psychological problems. Only after a period of warming up, or in a mood of jest, does some bitterness come to the surface— such as their complaints about the differences in freedom to call in late. It is quite apparent that for most, the ability to block off resentment against men is necessary in order to function smoothly in the hospital situation.

As opposed to medical school or the residency, the female intern receives little protection from department heads, attendants, fac-

[8] Report of a Civil Service order, Washington *Daily News* (ca. 1935), quoted in "The American female," *Harper's Magazine* (October, 1962), p. 132.

ulty, or other staff. This personal attention which sustained her and gave her occasional lifts during medical school no longer exists, and she must operate alone. Particularly in a rotating internship (although to some extent in a straight one also), she will be shifted from one service to another, and there is little chance for her to form any lasting relationships with superiors.

Two other groups must be dealt with extensively during the internship: nursing and paramedical staff, and the patients themselves. Some women are afraid in the beginning that they will not be able to give orders freely to the nurses, and male physicians wait with amusement for the first signs of rebellion against women doctors who cannot use seduction to get their way. "The men always think we're going to have trouble," reflected an intern, "but in many cases the nurses are nicer to us *because* we're women." Older nurses often maintain a protective, motherly attitude towards the women on the house staff which, although mixed with bantering, is still helpful in its support. A woman intern who had been on her feet without rest all weekend complained to a nurse that her ankles were quite painfully swollen. "Perhaps you're also starting your period.—Oh, but women physicians don't ovulate, do they?" said the nurse, who then went off to find the girl some relief for her ankles.

In her contact with patients, the woman intern invariably comes up against some who think *all* women must necessarily be nurses. Several interns told of completing a physical and hearing from the patient: "And now, when can I see the doctor?" Patients—particularly of the older age group—who see their first woman physician, make such statements as, "Now I've seen everything!" It can be an uncomfortable few minutes for a woman in her first encounter with a patient's resistance. "It's a matter of your own self-confidence. If you can convey your professionalism to the patient, he'll soon forget you're a woman," said an intern, who confessed she had nearly resigned one of her first patients to a male colleague when he steadfastly refused to believe she was the doctor.

Special Programs for Mother Interns

As the medical situation stands now, there is little one can do with an M.D. degree without taking an internship. Whatever personal strain it may cause a young person, this period can only become increasingly difficult with age. All older women doctors recommend that it be taken immediately after graduation from medical school. This is easier said than done when the woman is pregnant or has small children to look after. Despite the conscientious drive to be treated equally and to perform as well as and as devotedly as the men, some mother-physicians have had to make the choice between dropping out of medicine altogether or finding a program which would accept their limited participation. As of 1965, the *Directory of Approved Internships and Residencies* has sanctioned part-time internships " . . . in the case of female graduates of medical schools who have obligations, especially to those of dependent children, which prevent them from engaging in full-time internship activities." The 1966 *Directory* states:

> The Council does not wish to discourage the appointment of qualified female physicians to part-time internships, provided the responsible program director is able to arrange a program which meets the educational needs of the trainee and provided its total extent results in the sum of clinical experience and responsibilities acquired by an intern on a normal schedule. Such a part-time plan must be fair to the other interns and fully compatible with the hospital's training program and responsibilities in the care of patients.[9]

So far, only a few such programs have been established, and most of them have been instituted by individual request. The reception by the women themselves has been unenthusiastic, their general feeling being that it is exactly this period which "separates the men from the boys," and that they will be demonstrating their unsuitability by taking an easier route. One woman doctor ex-

---

[9] *Directory of Approved Internships and Residencies* (American Medical Association, 1966), p. 125.

pressed this point of view in the following terms: "The best way to get women discriminated against is to offer them the 'privilege' of a watered-down program. Such efforts cannot help but result in dissatisfaction among male house officers and poor training for the women who feel like a fifth wheel."

At French Hospital in New York City, a program was offered two years ago to take four women doctors with children in the place of two full-time interns. It was proposed that the mothers undergo a 24-month internship, with three months off each year. At any one time, one of them would be working two out of three nights and weekends but no week days, two would work week days only, and the fourth would be off duty altogether. At the end of a month, or whenever convenient, they would shift duties. In this way, there would always be complete coverage of two intern positions, and regular interns at the hospital would not suffer. Although the mothers would be working full-time, the salary offered them was $4,200 (that of the other interns at the hospital) since it was realized that a person could not be expected to live on much less. The program was scheduled to cost an additional $14,000 a year (including benefits), which the hospital felt was worth the expense if it could help qualified women to remain in medicine. Although it was never publicized nationally, hospital administrators went to several medical schools on the Eastern seaboard to offer it to their women students. Part-time internships were never put into effect at French Hospital, since no more than two women wanted to become involved at any one time.[10]

[10] In Seattle, Dr. David Shurtleff, Associate Professor of Pediatrics at the University of Washington Medical School, found much the same reaction. In 1963, he tried to set up residencies in which women could take three years to complete a two-year program. His idea was to accept at least two or three residents and allow them to work out schedules according to their individual needs, while still receiving the same training and donating the same service. Although the program was never advertised officially, Dr. Shurtleff told every woman about it who applied to him for a pediatric residency. In the four years that he has offered the program, there have been no applicants. The women have said they do not want what might be called second-rate training. All of them stated that they could handle a

During this period, however, one woman—the mother of five children—was allowed to take her internship in the hospital with greatly reduced night and weekend duty. Although this woman was overly conscientious, often staying on because of staff shortage when she actually had been given permission to return to her family, her "privileged" status caused resentment among the rest of the staff, and the hospital administration decided that it could not repeat such privileges on an individual basis.[11]

Another hospital, Bronx Lebanon, which requires alternate nights and weekend duty from its regular internship staff, has allowed mother-interns to work as little as one night a week and one weekend a month. There are now three women in this program, two taking a rotating internship and another taking one in pediatrics. Three other mothers have completed their internship under this system. Dr. Milton Goodfriend, Director of the program, states, "At times there is resentment by the men, but after they get to know the women this lessens. They need time off too, to help if their wives are sick, for instance, and they get it without any problems."[12]

Although administrative backing of a special "mother's program" may be able to influence the reactions of other interns in the hospital, it is obvious that giving dispensations to one group in a situation which is extremely demanding cannot help but cause resentment. Women in medicine may have to learn to cope with the hostility until the time that easier treatment is extended to all interns, regardless of sex. This is preferable to the misplaced pride of some women, who would waste their service to the profession altogether rather than face the humiliation of less than complete dedication.

"regular residency" as well as the men. From a personal communication, reported at the Macy Conference on Women for Medicine (October, 1966).

[11] Personal communication with Ralph Hertz, M.D., French Hospital, New York (April, 1967).

[12] Personal communication with Milton Goodfriend, M.D., Bronx Lebanon Hospital, Bronx, New York (April, 1967).

VIII

SPECIALIZATION AND THE RESIDENCY

With the internship over, physicians who decide to specialize—and an increasing proportion do—enter the last stage of their training, the three to five years of residency. A large proportion of both men and women are by now married; many have children. According to a follow-up study of physicians graduating in the class of 1956, 63 per cent of the women were married before completing residency or fellowship training, and more than one-third of all children born to these women were born before their mothers completed training. (Eighty per cent of the sample of male graduates of the class of 1956 were married before the end of their residency or fellowship training, and 60 per cent of all of their children were born before they had completed training.)[1] It is with the end of the internship that those women who continue in their profession begin to plan seriously for their dual roles as women and professionals.

The Choice of a Specialty

The choice of a specialty is contingent on several factors. Large differences exist among the various specialties and hospital programs in the competition for positions, the length of training involved, skills demanded, amount of in-hospital time required, and the general flexibility of the training program. In addition, looking ahead to the end of the residency period, there are differences in

[1] Lee Powers, Harry Wiesenfelder, and Rexford C. Parmelee, "Practice patterns of women and men physicians," Preliminary Report (October, 1966), Tables 4–B and 5.

the possible arrangements for a scheduled practice once certification is gained. Another factor is the general image of the specialty and its acceptance of women.

Of the three fields which together claim over 50 per cent of all women physicians receiving certification—pediatrics, internal medicine, and psychiatry—two have achieved the image of being "women's specialties." By far the most popular field among women is pediatrics (see Table 8–1). The source of its attraction is obvious: it is simply a field in which women feel comfortable and know they can excel. A pediatric resident in a small hospital writes: "Having your own children helps, because you understand a mother's problems. And a pediatrician has to be able to deal with *mothers* along with, and as frequently as, with children." This resident adds: "A woman's voice is also less frightening to a child, who will often scream whenever a male physician approaches." An older physician who raised five children while maintaining a position in pediatric cardiology in a large teaching hospital remarked, "It's helpful just to be a parent—of either sex; but simply being a parent gives you a great deal of insight into working with the mothers and fathers of the children."

Since pediatrics is the most obvious field for using the special skills of women, and since their value to the specialty has been proven, they have received warm acceptance by most department heads. Dr. Charles Janeway, Physician-in-Chief at Children's Hospital in Boston, reports of his part-time mother-residents in pediatrics:

> These women, who already have experience with child-rearing in their own homes, have proven to be particularly effective pediatric residents in dealing with many of the emotional and social problems which form such a large component of the patients we see in our pediatric clinic. In addition, they are good doctors, stable people, with more maturity and good judgment than one would expect in younger physicians.[2]

[2] Personal communication with Charles Janeway, M.D. (April, 1967).

TABLE 8–1. PERCENTAGE OF WOMEN AND MEN RECEIVING
CERTIFICATION BY SPECIALTY BOARDS

Specialty board	Women		Men	
	No.	*(per cent)*	No.	*(per cent)*
Pediatrics	152	33.6	79	10.6
Psychiatry and Neurology	62	13.7	55	7.4
Internal Medicine	45	10.0	127	17.0
Anesthesiology	41	9.1	30	4.0
Pathology	39	8.6	34	4.6
Obstetrics and Gynecology	36	8.0	68	9.1
Radiology	28	6.2	55	7.4
Preventive Medicine	14	3.1	19	2.5
Ophthalmology	9	2.0	32	4.3
General Surgery	7	1.6	116	15.5
Dermatology	7	1.5	25	3.4
Physical Medicine and Rehabilitation	4	.9	3	.4
Orthopedic Surgery	4	.9	31	4.2
Otolaryngology	2	.4	24	3.2
Plastic Surgery	2	.4	8	1.1
Neurological Surgery	—	—	8	1.1
Thoracic Surgery	—	—	17	2.2
Urology	—	—	15	2.0
Total certifications	452	100.0	746	100.0
Number of physicians certified	445	33.3	721	45.5
Number of physicians not certified	891	66.7	863	54.5
Total physicians	1336	100.0	1584	100.0

Source: A preliminary report, "Practice patterns of women and men physicians," by Lee Powers, Harry Wiesenfelder, and Rexford C. Parmelee (October 14, 1966), Table 22.

The few scattered part-time residency programs which have been set up throughout the country have been mainly in pediatrics and psychiatry, two fields which are concerned with the mother-child relationship and which take a large number of women physicians.

Like pediatrics, psychiatry deals with the growth process of the individual. (In interviews, women physicians often give this as a specific reason for choosing this specialty.) Women have traditionally been considered sensitive to the emotional aspects of interpersonal situations. The same qualities which make them more "field-oriented" in psychological tests may also give them the continued desire to help another person work out his or her problems. And women are often able to keep their egos in the background and not to compete as directly, so that the clashes of will which sometimes destroy the physician-patient relationship in psychotherapy may occur less frequently with female than with male therapists.

Maternal feelings can also be of great value in treating the emotionally disturbed patient—be he child or adult. In fact, the field of child psychiatry has been dominated from the first by contributions of women (Anna Freud, Melanie Klein, Lauretta Bender, Margaret Mahlor, Sybil Escalona, etc.). In the practical sphere, the minimal amount of night and weekend duty during the residency and the possibility for flexible scheduling once training is over make psychiatry one of the most attractive specialties for women physicians with families.[3]

The comfort which a woman feels in practicing her specialty is largely dependent on the resolution of any conflict which might exist between her sexual and professional roles. John Kosa and Robert E. Cocker, in a study of women in "feminine" specialties such as pediatrics, psychiatry, and public health, outlines the sources of role conflict and their common means of resolution:

> If we consider the problem of females as the minority sex in medicine, we may theoretically outline three main areas of role conflict as well as professional procedure to cope with those conflicts. It is reasonable to assume that: (1) the professional role tends to impose limitations upon the full realization of the female role; (2) the female role tends to limit the full realization of the professional role; and, in addition; (3) female practitioners face particular difficulties in assuming those professional duties which are more or less incompatible with female tasks. While the three areas of conflict are, to a great extent, overlapping and make it difficult, or impossible, to restrict the role conflict to one area only,

[3] One cannot overlook the fact that child psychiatry requires the maximum number of years of residency. This can be a serious barrier for the married woman with children, though not necessarily an obstacle for a single woman.

women doctors tend to manage their professional careers by selecting for work those fields of medicine and that type of practice which are least likely to offer work duties incompatible with the female task.[4]

It is interesting that many women enter public health after having practiced pediatrics during the earlier part of their lives. Both fields are concerned with the preventive side of medicine; and public health provides opportunities for organizing medical care to improve the health of a larger segment of the population than can come to a private office. Public health work also offers regular hours and a salary—not as easily available in pediatric practice. Kosa and Cocker state that, when selecting public health ". . . the female physician expects an alleviation of those limitations that the sex role puts upon the full performance of the professional role and, at the same time, a reduction of the possible conflict centering around the entrepreneurial role and free competition with members of the opposite sex."[5] A Boston physician taking a part-time residency in public health writes about the way in which she was able to secure this privileged schedule:

> Because of my husband's position, we are permanently settled in this area so that I am a 'good investment' for the field of public health in Massachusetts, and also I was elected to the honor society at the Harvard School of Public Health. In addition, [as the public health official told her] because of the unique advantages of public health, it tends to attract highly qualified women (men with the same qualifications are free to enter any field of medicine, and, therefore, are more widely dispersed through all fields). He felt that the sacrifices that had to be made for qualified women were repaid in the long run.

In contrast to the previously mentioned specialties, internal medicine cannot be considered to attract women through either its

[4] John Kosa and Robert E. Cocker, "The female physician in public health, and reconciliation of the sex and professional roles," *Sociology and Social Research* 49, no. 3 (April, 1965):295.

[5] *Ibid.*, p. 304.

"feminine" image or its possibilities for scheduling. Internal medicine is a highly competitive, extremely demanding specialty. With the disappearance of the general practitioner, specialists in internal medicine have taken over much of their work in addition to the regular specialty practice. Among many physicians, internal medicine is considered to offer the greatest amount of intellectual challenge and possibilities for varied practice. A woman internist can be sure to feel in the thick of medicine.

A strong rationale for permitting women to become physicians in the nineteenth century was that they would take care of the "feminine ailments" of those of their sex who would otherwise have done without treatment. Although twentieth-century women have become less Victorian in their attitudes towards male physicians, there are some who continue to feel that members of their own sex will be more understanding in dealing with such problems.

A young woman who was entering a residency in obstetrics-gynecology expressed the desire to bring a "female" approach to the profession. Extensive pelvic surgery, such as a hysterectomy or oophorectomy, might have been avoided in some cases, she felt, had the physician been a woman and more capable of empathizing. She was not yet married, and so did not have to think in terms of regular hours or flexible scheduling during the next few years, which might have restricted her choice to fields other than Ob-Gyn (babies can be born at any time, day or night). Since women are also, quite naturally, attracted to the birth process, it seems likely that they will continue to enter obstetrics-gynecology: some of the pleasures and gratifications to be found in modern obstetrics are not entirely different from those of the traditional midwife.

Reasons for selecting a specialty may vary from woman to woman within any one field. Although scheduling can be an important incentive—pathology, radiology, anesthesiology, dermatology, and ophthamology provide excellent scheduling opportunities —the sheer attraction of a field can obviously convince a woman to make sacrifices in favor of her interest. One unmarried, energetic, and lively redhead had chosen anesthesiology because she felt that women should stay out of the "men's fields." She wanted a specialty which she would be able to schedule around her future husband's needs, but she also loved the excitement of the operating room. When I met her, she had just spent the night helping to deliver half-a-dozen babies: her enthusiasm for the work often kept her in the hospital far more than her reasoned-out desire for a scheduled life would have permitted.

The particular chief of service may also be important in a choice of specialty. A married physician with two children switched from a pediatric residency to pediatric radiology after a year because of her "respect for the radiology department head." She felt that the residents in radiology were much happier as a group than those in pediatrics, due largely to the atmosphere created by the department head.

Two women dermatologists provide an interesting contrast in the reasons given for choosing a particular specialty. One had entered her residency after a demanding internship during which, she said, "I really think I might have damaged my children." The irregularity of her schedule had kept her whole family on edge, and she was determined to find a field in which her husband and children could expect her to be with them in the evenings. Only as she went along in the dermatology program did she find, happily, an interest in the field.

Another gave a more personal reason. "I had overt anxiety about making an error that would lead to a patient's death, and this influenced my choice of dermatology as a specialty."[6] At the time when the second woman was questioned, she was doing research part-time under an NIH Public Health Service Grant, and looked forward to the next years in which she hoped she would be able to give up medicine altogether. Having conquered some of her fears through psychotherapy, she went on to realize that medicine had been a mistake for her, and she decided to give her creative im-

[6] Quoted in Eli Ginzberg and Alice M. Yohalem, *Educated American Women: Self-Portraits* (New York: Columbia University Press, 1966), p. 162.

pulses, which had been "stifled" when younger, a chance through full-time painting.

Dividing up the turf in a marriage of two physicians, or in a family of two or more doctors, can be an important reason for the choice of one's specialty. Sometimes this is merely sweeping a problem under the rug. A woman physician who married a fellow student during medical school had made an agreement with him that she would not go into psychiatry—which he wanted to enter—because the competition would be too direct. Instead, she planned to work in pediatrics, a field in which she thought she could become interested. An ironic solution to the conflict occurred, however. They divorced at the end of medical school, and she was able to switch back to psychiatry. The last indirect news she had heard of him was that he had entered an entirely different area—computer designing for medicine.

Even when two members of a family share the same specialty, it is common to hear from the woman, "He does the research, and I do the practice," or "We're really interested in totally different aspects of the field."[7]

The difficulty of coping with male-female competition may be an important reason why certain specialties have remained predominately male, while others have attracted women. The women themselves, of course, have played a part in maintaining this division. For her thesis on "The Professional Status of Women in Medicine," Josephine Williams interviewed male and female medical students about the specialties that they felt were particularly suited to men or women. She found that fewer women conceded male superiority in most specialties than the proportion of men who claimed it; however, both sexes agreed that surgery was a man's field. In addition, women and men agreed more often on the ability of women to perform well in professions which they both felt had

---

[7] On the other hand, some couples function as medical partners, and the work of close associates in a laboratory has been known to end at times in marriage—one method of seeing that the information stays in the same hands.

less prestige: anesthesiology, obstetrics-gynecology, pediatrics, etc.[8]

At the Macy Conference on Women for Medicine, Dr. Edithe Levit, Assistant Director of the National Board of Medical Examiners, made a sensible protest against confining women physicians to the careers they have traditionally taken:

> Fifty years ago, we would have heard the well-known phrase, "The woman's place is in the home." Now that we have allowed her to move into the medical world, I'm afraid we're saying, "The woman's place is in pediatrics or child psychiatry, etc." I submit that we can no more say that the woman, because she is a woman, is better suited for pediatrics than she is for surgery, any more than we can say that a man, simply because he is a man, is better suited for surgery than pediatrics.

Through a combination of choice and prejudice against them, women are scarcely represented in certain specialties. Ophthalmology, orthopedic, thoracic, plastic, and neurological surgery show few female physicians certified by their boards (16 per cent of the certified male physicians sampled listed their specialty as general surgery, in contrast to less than 2 per cent of the women). Fields such as urology, gastroenterology, and aviation medicine are almost devoid of women. While there is a good reason why women do not select orthopedic surgery (which is physically strenuous) or aviation medicine, which remains a predominately male field, many of the surgical specialties could, as far as skills and interests are concerned, become equally important women's areas.

In order to enter a specialty, one must win the approval of the head of the residency program, and it is here that women have sometimes faced an unconquerable barrier. The limitation of residency positions in the surgical specialties and the popularity and high demand for these places puts the bargaining power in the hands of the department heads. Over 90 per cent of the residencies in neurological surgery, ophthalmology, orthopedic surgery, otolaryngology, and plastic surgery are filled each year, compared to only

[8] Josephine J. Williams, "The professional status of women in medicine" (unpublished Ph.D. dissertation, Department of Sociology, University of Chicago, 1949).

one-half to three-fourths in some other specialties.[9] Department heads in these surgical specialties feel that they would rather pick from the best male candidates than take a chance on a woman. (Although women have averaged only a fraction of a year less than men in their amount of graduate training—2.26 as opposed to 2.55 over the past 30 years[10]—their higher rate of mobility and even their temporary withdrawal to bear children can create difficulties in the administration of the departments in which they serve.)

A graduate of a top medical school, who was taking her residency in psychiatry, complained that she had actually wanted to become an ophthalmologist and had spent summers doing research on the eye, but had been forced to change because of the overt prejudice she had found among heads of the programs where she applied. One physician said he had never bothered to interview women, while another had told her, "Wait until the war escalates; we couldn't possibly consider you now." With only 4,800 board-certified ophthalmologists serving apopulation of 193 million, department heads of programs in ophthalmology feel that they must get the most man-hours out of their graduates. The alternate solution of increasing the number of residency positions and trained ophthalmologists will have to come about, and when it does, women should be well suited to the specialty.

A woman physician who had succeeded in entering a residency in plastic surgery remarked, "It's the only field where you can be 30 years old and still get spanked every day." But, as she herself realized, when a woman insists on competing with a man for a most desirable position, she will likely be choosing a life in which there is no rest from suspicious tests of her ability. "If you decide to become a surgeon," remarked this woman, "You'd better be sure

[9] *Directory of Approved Internships and Residencies* (American Medical Association, 1966), p. 8.

[10] Powers, Wiesenfelder, and Parmelee, "Practice patterns of women and men physicians," Table 21.

you can carry through without having to ask for any dispensations for your feminine needs."

Being skillful at their own protection, few contemporary women actually come face-to-face with a door locked against them. Most veer off into the more acceptable and accepting specialties, without even a wistful look at those fields which might have spurned them. There is little of the suffragette attitude which once inspired women physicians to enter a specialty simply because their sex was not represented. With this new casual attitude, however, inroads can be made. Certain general changes will increase the area of operations for women physicians: (1) the further centering of medicine in clinics and hospitals, leading to regular work hours; and (2) a general relaxation on all candidates of service demanded during the internship and residency training. As these occur, there will probably be little reason for prejudice against women or hesitation on their part to enter freely the specialties they desire.

The Married Resident

Residency programs run from two to five years—the shortest in pediatrics, and the longest in child psychiatry and the surgical sub-specialties. Residents live outside the hospital but spend one or more nights a week on call, depending upon their specialty, the rules of the individual hospital department, and their degree of training. In a good residency program, these years follow the internship in a smooth continuum of increased responsibility for patient care.

For the woman resident with no new outside duties, the years will probably be easier and more pleasant than the time spent during the internship. Although the same sources of difficulties with colleagues and staff still exist, the decrease in pressure and competition makes these take a far milder form, becoming in some cases hardly noticeable. The woman is further along in her training, and having chosen a specialty which suits her, can with mounting confidence put down potentially aggravating situations. In a field such as surgery, which has few women, the female resident may still feel on trial during much of her working day. However, in other specialties, after an initial period of proving herself, the woman resident can usually operate unself-consciously, fulfilling her assignments with security and the knowledge that she is becoming a specialist in the field.

The majority of married women residents adjust their personal lives around a regular residency schedule, and ask for very few special privileges. However, the burden of responsibilities pulling in two directions—home and hospital—often causes the fear that one or the other activity will suffer. In the past when conflicts arose, women took leaves from medicine rather than deny their family's pressing needs. But as part-time positions for women became available throughout the working world, women physicians began to have the courage to ask for professional arrangements which fit their duties as wives and mothers. This section is devoted to the particular problems of wife-and-mother residents, a group which—with the lowering of the average age for marriage and for child-bearing—has come to comprise an increasing proportion of the women in training.

In medicine, as in other demanding fields, a woman's life-cycle and her dependency upon the geographic location of her husband conflict with responsibilities to her profession. Margaret Mead has written that "our academic tradition was initially designed by and for the celibate, the monk, the occasional nun, a kind of sexless life in which activities of the intellect were joined with a disavowal of the flesh and a denial of the body. The academic world is fundamentally hostile, by tradition, to those acts of femininity which involve childbearing."[11] Even where the "hostility" may not be an emotional factor, the institutionalized requirements of medicine remain at odds with those of wifehood and motherhood.

[11] Margaret Mead, "Gender in the Honors program," *Newsletter of the Inter-University Committee on the Superior Student* (May, 1961), pp. 4–5.

A department chairman expressed the discomfort characteristic of those in his position: "A man feels particularly frustrated in trying to meet these arguments [of moving and pregnancy], because they are particularly feminine arguments, and if you try to hold the residents to a contract, then you are arguing against motherhood and all those things, and it is a psychologically bad point of view for a male department chairman to take." However, since only around 80 per cent of the residency positions throughout the country are filled each year (and of these, 29 per cent are held by foreign graduates,[12] chiefs of staff have taken women candidates even when their personal feelings might have swayed them against them.

One of the first reactions of some department heads to the subject of women residents is their annoyance at having been left without a staff member because a woman did not keep to her contract. If the female resident is married to another graduate physician, a good deal of effort is expended to ensure that the two will be able to train together, thus decreasing the chance of moves. A dean of one school may spend several hours making long-distance telephone calls to work out arrangements for a resident-physician. The birth of a child, of course, is a more difficult problem to solve. A woman may voluntarily return to work within a week or so after delivery—and many do. However, if she has decided to bring up the child herself during the first few years, hospital administrators have traditionally felt there is little that can be arranged to hold her.

This has made the relationship between chiefs of service and female residents a sensitive one. Department heads have learned the value of taking women onto their staff, and acknowledge that the work these female residents give to the job is often of the highest caliber. "The women I've dealt with have been a remarkably competent, hard-working lot," observed one chief. But it is all the more difficult to come to terms with the loss of a woman resident—

[12] *Directory of Approved Internships and Residencies,* p. 6.

the very same woman, in some cases, whose stability and hard work
had won him over despite prejudice or misgivings, and whose de-
sertion comes as a personal betrayal. A chief of service jocularly
characterized the vulnerability of his position in the following
words: "If she's single, she'll get married; if she's married, she'll
have a baby; and if she's got both a husband *and* a child, she'll
leave to get a divorce."

The psychological difficulty of the situation affects the women
also, and causes them to operate at times in a devious way. Sensing
how much was at stake, a woman resident told me she fearfully
held off warning her chairman of a pending departure. When she
had applied to the program he had accepted her hesitantly, telling
her of the bad luck he had had with other women who left him
in the lurch after only a year. Now her husband had received a
position in another city, and she passed her supervisor's office day
after day, trying to get the courage to tell him she would have to
leave. "I just never believed it would happen a year ago," she shook
her head with embarrassment.

One means of decreasing the possibility of withdrawal by women
residents involves a concession on the part of their department
heads (as well as the American Specialty Boards) to a less demanding schedule. Such a concession, however, could in time make an
important contribution to medical womanpower.

Within the limitations of his responsibilities to the appropriate
specialty board—and the actual rulings set down by the boards
leave room for much variation—the department chairman has great
freedom in establishing the atmosphere and day-to-day structure
of his residency program. Because of their authority, department
heads have often been able to make special arrangements for
mother-residents—delivery leave, reduced night and weekend
duty, etc. As with the part-time internships, nearly all of the exist-
ing special arrangements for mother-residents have been worked
out on an individual basis between the woman and her department
head, after which approval has been solicited from the specialty
board. Of course, chiefs of departments are not uniformly receptive

to the idea of using part-time residents: the cost is usually a little higher to the hospital, a reduction in service may result, or the training may simply not be deemed sufficient by the board. Residency programs in psychiatry—which has had more part-time women residents working to pass the boards than any other specialty—also have the advantage of needing less night and weekend service of residents, as opposed to training programs in specialties which deal more frequently with emergencies—internal medicine or obstetrics-gynecology, for instance.

In the spring of 1967, the major specialty boards supplied information on their policies regarding part-time residencies for women with dependent children. Table 8–2 shows these specialties, the usual length of training and hours demanded under a regular residency program, and the decision of the boards regarding part-time training.

It is possible that more boards might be amenable if an excellent program were proposed, but not having seen one, they hesitate to take a stand. Complicating the issue is the fact that the amount of night and weekend training necessary for board certification has never been rigidly set in any specialty, and the time demanded of a resident physician has undergone consistent relaxation in the past years, irrespective of the needs of women medical graduates. If an open statement were made that women could be adequately prepared with reduced—or without—night and weekend experience, this would present an even greater challenge to the present system of keeping resident physicians on duty several nights a week and every other weekend.

The attempt to give reduced training over a longer period is relatively recent and will have to be tried out more extensively before everyone concerned can feel more at ease with it. The reaction of President Leymaster of Woman's Medical College to part-time training for women residents is not surprising, considering the newness of the concept in the medical profession: "I confess," he remarked at the Macy Conference, after hearing of several such programs, "that until recently I tended to minimize the problems

TABLE 8–2.   A COMPARISON OF THE USUAL RESIDENCY SERVICE AND
SPECIALTY BOARD POLICY REGARDING PART-TIME TRAINING

Specialty	Usual length of residency training	Regular duty for resident	Board policy regarding part-time residencies
Anesthesiology	3 years	in-hospital, on-at-night	part-time accepted
Dermatology	3 years	usually out-patient	part-time accepted[1]
Internal medicine	3 years	in-hospital, on-at-night	very occasionally, on an individual basis
Obstetrics-Gynecology	3 or more years	in-hospital, on-at-night	not accepted
Ophthalmology	3 years	usually out-patient	not accepted[1]
Pathology	4 years	in-hospital, but schedule possible	not accepted
Pediatrics	2 years or more	in-hospital, on-at-night	very occasionally on an individual basis[2]
Psychiatry-Neurology	3 years (or more for child psychiatry)	in-hospital, but schedule possible	half-time accepted
Public health	2 years	usually out-patient	part-time accepted
Radiology	3 years	in-hospital, but schedule possible	very occasionally, on an individual basis
General surgery	4 or more years	in-hospital, on-at-night	not accepted

[1] The possibility of receiving preceptorships in the private office of a staff member in dermatology or opthalmology may give women an added chance to work out scheduling which fits their needs, although this is not considered the most desirable means of gaining training.

[2] The Board has also certified "broken residencies" in which the women can take off 3-to-6 months at a time.

of the formal internship and residency programs, and tended to pay a great deal more attention to what I call the retraining of women after they have been out of active practice for a few years because of children."

Since part-time residencies and retraining programs are the two alternates available to women with children, it will be helpful, before going further, to compare these approaches. So far, two centers have become involved in retraining women physicians: one, the Woman's Medical College in Philadelphia, and another, the Presbyterian Hospital Medical Center in San Francisco. The Woman's Medical College Retraining Center is intended as an integral part of the medical school. Still in its pilot stage, it will attempt to renovate the training of women physicians who have been out of the profession for five or more years. The women will receive programs individually tailored to their needs and future goals. Training is estimated to take eighteen months, on a some what more than half-time basis.

The program at the Presbyterian Hospital Medical Center in San Francisco was established in 1966 to provide fellowships from six months to a year for women who wish to return to medical practice after a period of inactivity of ten or more years. Coordinators of the program favor women who have achieved Board-eligible status. Those women who have not achieved Board-eligible status are offered a rotation through internal medicine, pediatrics, office gynecology, minor surgery, and emergency work, with schedules to fit individual plans. Stipends for full-time trainees follow the U.S. Public Health Service fellowship rule: $5,000 per year as basic payment, and $500 for each year of post-doctoral training (internship, residency, and fellowship). An additional $500 is available for each dependent if the applicant is the sole support; $3,600 of the stipend is tax-exempt.

These two programs are experimenting with an exceedingly difficult and important problem: how to bring a woman's professional training up-to-date in fields which have changed drastically in the last decade. If successful, they could bring back into practice a large proportion of the women who have become inactive after graduation. Even if only half of the women classified as "inactive"[13] could be coaxed out of their homes, their productivity would exceed that of the graduating classes of half a dozen medical schools.

The importance of retraining programs in the immediate future is obvious: they will bring manpower to overly taxed services and give a second chance to women who have either dropped out entirely or who are working at jobs far below their ability and interest. As an example, a thirty-five-year-old woman who completed her internship and then stopped training to have four children in succession writes, "I'd like to look forward to a 20-to-40-hour week in some field in about three years. But after a ten-year lapse, I'm unprepared. I work a bit with Bloodmobile, and that's no preparation for anything." If a Center is in her area when this woman is ready to retrain, she can go on to give at least thirty more years to medicine.

Still, the retraining approach in medicine has some severe drawbacks. The organization of ten years in the profession, then ten or so in withdrawal and, hopefully, the return to it again at the age of thirty-five or forty, is particularly wasteful in scientific fields where the late twenties and early thirties are the most creative years.[14] Women who have dropped out entirely for a substantial period rarely return to operate with the same energy and efficiency as those who have remained continuously in the profession.

In an article entitled, "Women in Science; Why So Few?" Alice Rossi sums up the case against retraining professional women:

> During the last five years there has been a mushrooming of centers for counseling and retraining older women who wish to re-

[13] As of December 31, 1965, 2,572 women were classified by the AMA as inactive—out of a total of 19,526 women physicians. Since there is no definition for the term "inactive," however, these data are not very exact. (Statistics provided by the National Center for Health Statistics, U.S. Public Health Service, based on individual physician's records from the American Medical Association [December 31, 1965].)

[14] Harvey C. Lehman, *Age and Achievement* (Princeton, N.J.: Princeton University Press, 1963).

turn to professional employment. I think there is a danger that by thus institutionalizing the withdrawal-and-return pattern of college-educated women, we may reduce even further the likelihood that women will enter the top professions. Older women who have not worked for many years may be retrained and contribute significantly to personnel shortages at the lower professional levels as laboratory assistants, technical writers, nurses, and school teachers, but only rarely as doctors, full-fledged scientists, and engineers. Not only is training for such fields a long and difficult process, but the pace of technological and scientific knowledge has been so rapid that even those who remain in these fields have difficulty keeping up, let alone those who return to advanced training after a 10-year break.[15]

It is estimated that the turnover in medical knowledge is now five years: unless continually revitalized by reading and contact with other physicians, a person five years out of the profession can only give outmoded medical care. With the increasingly rapid advances, even a physician practicing full-time will soon have to spend one half-day a week or the equivalent reading and hearing lectures in order to maintain his professional competence. This makes retraining a huge proposition. Dr. Leymaster estimates that his retraining program at Woman's Medical will cost $8,000–$10,000 per student per year, which is more expensive than training a medical student.[16] When one considers the reduced capabilities of the woman due to her age and years out of practice, such a Center does not seem to be an economical proposition. The great need for physicians and the large group of women doctors now out of the field because of the rigidity of graduate training justifies such an expense. But hopefully, with increased opportunities for part-time work and training throughout the child-rearing years, the next generation of women doctors will not have to face this problem in such great numbers.

The women themselves who re-enter medicine after a period of

[15] Alice Rossi, "Women in science; why so few?" *Science* 48 (May, 1965):1199.
[16] Personal communication with Glen R. Leymaster, M.D., May, 1967.

withdrawal consistently report they would have preferred to keep their hand in the profession rather than to start again at the age of thirty-five or forty. A pediatrician who had dropped out at the birth of her second child after a year of residency, returned for part-time training ten years later when a hospital in the community offered for the first time a residency that allowed greater flexibility. This program did not offer retraining courses. She had no trouble with well-baby care in the out-patient clinic, she said, but was at a disadvantage when it came to complex diagnostic and therapeutic procedures. Her difficulties were enhanced by the fact that her resident duties included advising young doctors who were "fresh from the books, fresh from their internship, and just plain fresh!" After a few weeks of bluffing, she asked to be given rounds with the other interns until she had caught up—even though her hours would no longer be part-time.

Stories about similar cases of humility among women returning to medicine are common, and point to the fact that they work hard to come up to their own stringent standards. In general, women in special programs (part-time, retraining, or whatever) have a scrupulous sense of responsibility and are loath to exploit their favorable situation. If anything, they do not take advantage of the full opportunities offered them; but the knowledge that such freedom exists may help them through the rougher moments.

From the standpoint of adjustment and strain on the woman, part-time training immediately following the internship, or part-time practice until regular training is possible, would seem to be a less harrowing solution than retraining. A consideration of medical education costs shows that it is also more economical. When the salaries awarded to two part-time residents are prorated for the amount of hours worked, it costs the hospital little more than does a full-time resident—mainly the doubling of benefit expenses to two employees. Teaching expenses are far lower than those estimated in retraining programs, since the women need no more extensive training than their full-time male and female colleagues.

A special program for mother-residents in psychiatry at the New

York Medical College points to some major advantages over re-training programs, although it is only a halfway-house between the standard full-time and a genuinely part-time schedule. The program was first set up in 1962 by Drs. Alfred Freedman and Harold Kaplan, when Dr. Kaplan's wife was struggling to complete her training under the regular program. The two men decided to institute a pilot program which would help her and others like her to go through with less difficulty. They received approval from the American Board for a three-year residency in general psychiatry which would be spread out over four years, and were able to obtain financing from the National Institute of Mental Health. The mother-residents receive a base salary of $5,640 (the same as their male colleagues), which is prorated for the time worked. The women receive a maximum of three months off a year for their family, taken whenever they wish; thus, their salary comes to a little over $4,000 per year. Participants in the program —there have been twenty women so far—work a nine-to-five day, five days a week, which was a major qualification for receiving the NIMH grant. However, night and weekend duty in the New York program are reduced to the minimum required for satisfactory training. The mother-physicians also have the understanding that if any emergency arises at home, a change in schedule can be arranged and will be accepted. The women often cover assignments for each other in family emergencies. Scheduling is flexible enough to have enabled a woman with eleven children to be salvaged by the program!

A major difference between the New York program and the part-time residencies worked out by individual mothers and their department heads is the "institutionalization of flexibility." While in every hospital a degree of flexibility is given to both male and female residents, there is a tendency for the men to resent any privileges a woman on the staff receives, and this makes the women reluctant to ask for any. At the New York Medical College, administrators sanction the program, giving it a stamp of legitimacy. If a man is at times called on to take over for a mother-resident, there is less resistance than would be the case in a hospital where one or two women had been singled out for special treatment. In an article on the mother's program, Dr. Harold Kaplan states, "The resistance of male doctors to 'pitching in' and assuming extra assignments when, for example, the mother-resident is on vacation, is nothing more than what they customarily do for their male peers regularly and without resentment. It is our observation that such problems are fundamentally administrator-induced rather than inherent in the young male doctor."[17]

As an interesting side-comment, Dr. Edith Shapiro, coordinator of the Psychiatric Training Program for mother-residents, reports that "Only one out of the twenty mothers has used her full three months of leave each summer while in the program. Three have taken a two-months' leave of absence each summer, and the rest have averaged only one month's leave each summer. All have taken three-to-four days off during the year . . . Except for the major blocks of time labeled leave, the mothers have actually taken less time off for personal business and less sick leave than is the average for the rest of the residency group."[18]

The mother-residents in the psychiatric training program are evaluated regularly and have done as well or better than the full-time residents, showing that they have not been noticeably deprived of any learning experiences. The full discharge of the service responsibility to the hospital is another, often raised question, but since the mother-residents total four years instead of three, the extra night and weekend duty is made up by the end of their training period.

A special feature of this program is that mother-residents take part in a weekly group-therapy discussion. In the cases where the mother-residents had been out for some time before entering the program, a good deal of energy is put into giving them the con-

[17] Harold Kaplan, "The crisis in the utilization of women physicians," *Medical Tribune* (July 29, 1964).

[18] Personal communication from Edith Shapiro, M.D., to Constance Smith, Dean of the Radcliffe Institute, October, 1966.

fidence to stick out the first hard months. Dr. Kaplan reports that he once had to bodily restrain a woman from walking out of her first exam. "She was so sure she could never pass it, but actually did quite well after she had calmed down," he said. The support of other women residents who have gone through the same adjustment is helpful.

In situations where part-time training is not formalized, encouragement by the other staff is even more important—and rarer to find. A pathologist who was able to work out special arrangements during her residency at Duke wrote, "It seems to me that there should be some recognition of the fact that most women who choose medicine will also want a home and family. As my chief often said, 'We need you, and any time you can give is to our advantage.' This attitude helped me a great deal, and I think it should and could be applied more widely. We are needed and wanted, but are not men, and our contributions should not be judged on that basis. We do not wish to compete with men, only to help them." The lack of this kind of support can completely change the nature of a woman's experience as a resident. Another respondent, who had not established any special part-time program but had had to take off at times because of family difficulties, answered a question about prejudice against women in the residency by saying, "I don't know about other women, but I, as the mother of a six-year-old daughter, was miserable the whole time. I had to fight for the smallest human consideration, and was punished by the lowest assignments."

One obstacle toward part-time programs for women has been finding sources to finance such experiments. An individual department chairman may allocate whatever funds he deems necessary to pay a half-time resident, if he has the permission of his hospital. When there have been only limited funds available, however, many women have had to accept annual salaries of $2,000; and for those who need household help, this makes working as a resident a costly venture. The programs of the National Institute of Health of the U.S. Public Health Service, which pay stipends to an increasing proportion of graduate physicians, still require that the grantee be in full-time training. Government loans permit recipients to be training half-time, but are simply not the answer for a graduate mother-physician who may already have debts and must give over most or all of her income to household help.

To ease this deadlock, in 1961 the Radcliffe Institute in Cambridge, Massachusetts, set up a special program to provide stipends to women for the pursuit of their medical training on a part-time basis. Radcliffe stipends range from $500 to $3,000 annually, but the average grant to physicians has been approximately $2,000, usually renewable for one year. The money is provided to pay for baby-sitters, household costs, transportation, texts, and other expenses. Where the income paid by the hospital to a half-time resident has been $6 to $8 a day, and a reliable baby-sitter's fee is $12 to $15, the Institute stipend has paid the difference. In addition, the Institute has helped to arrange for less than full-time residencies at hospitals in the Boston area, which until then had never made special accommodations for women physicians.

The first Radcliffe fellowship in medicine was given to Dr. Nancy Hendrie, who was also the first part-time resident in the history of Children's Hospital Medical Center. At the time she completed the program, Dr. Charles A. Janeway, Physician-in-Chief, remarked: "Judging by the great success we've had with Dr. Hendrie, . . . I hope we can continue to be flexible in adapting our programs to the needs of such able women."[19] Since that time, Children's Hospital Medical Center has accepted several more Radcliffe Institute women on a part-time basis.

As of July 1, 1966, the Institute medical trainees have been supported by funds from the Josiah Macy, Jr., Foundation, which made a four-year grant of $161,000 to the Institute to assist women medical graduates, especially in part-time training. In the first year,

[19] "Dr. Hendrie, HMC's first part-time resident," *News of the Children's Hospital Medical Center* (August, 1963), p. 10.

fourteen women were awarded Macy grants. The excerpts below, taken from the Institute's files on individual physicians, give an idea of the types of programs which these women have been able to work out in the Boston area through the Institute:

1. Two-year, half-time residency in child psychiatry at Massachusetts Mental Health Center, Children's Unit.
2. Two-year, half-time residency in child psychiatry at James Jackson Putnam Clinic.
3. One-year, full-time special course in pediatrics under the auspices of Harvard Medical School; one-year, half-time residency in pediatrics for ambulatory services, Children's Hospital Medical Center.
4. One-year, half-time residency in pediatrics at Children's Hospital Medical Center, to complete requirements for Board qualification.
5. Two year, half-time student at Harvard School of Public Health . . . degree of Master of Public Health (with honors).
6. Two-year, half-time residency in occupational medicine Har- Health Center.

The women at the Institute were at different stages in their residency training when they entered the part-time programs. The hospitals and fields in which they were training determined the actual schedule implied in the words "half-time." For one woman in pediatrics, half-time meant working four days and two nights, off at noon on Friday, with every other weekend on call; for a mother in occupational medicine, it meant working only three or four mornings a week.

There can be as many gradations of part-time programs as there are different needs of hospitals and mother-residents, and it would be foolish to recommend any one structure to cover all these situations. Indeed, this would defeat the point of part-time programs, whose purpose is to get out of a rigid system and to set up arrangements for individual circumstances. The only element advisable to special programs for women is that they be institutionalized in some way, whether by the hospital administration or an outside organization like the Radcliffe Institute. This cuts down on staff resentment, and the undertones of a "private deal," as well as the pressure and guilt feelings which mother-residents have to sustain.

At the Macy Conference on Women for Medicine, Constance Smith, Dean of the Institute, said: "We cannot know whether it is possible to train such women adequately on a part-time schedule unless we try some more flexible schedules. My proposal would be this: since women comprise approximately 6 per cent of those currently training in medicine, set up an experimental five-year program to administer 1 per cent or even one-half of 1 per cent of the present government training grants for less than full-time training. It is possible that men, too, will be interested in such grants, but it is certain that a number of women could benefit from such flexibility."

More and more fields in other sectors of society have made openings for part-time employment, either to women returning to work, to the over-65 population, or to men holding two jobs. In medicine itself, it is now possible to find part-time work in clinics, hospitals, or teaching. A growing number of male physicians hold half-time or three-fourths-time posts in research or academic medicine, while still practicing on the side. As this partitioning of work becomes more prevalent in other spheres through automation or staggered round-the-clock employment, the government will have to do something for all sources of manpower and womanpower which have been neglected because of their inability to work full-time. The part-time principle, which is already in effect in medical practice, can and should be extended backwards into the training period.

IX

MARRIAGE AND MEDICINE

A woman's goal, like that of men, is to develop a life style that uses her energies and capabilities in such a way that she functions in her various roles efficiently and productively, with sufficient integration among these roles to give her at least some personal satisfaction in each.[1]

Considered from this standpoint, women physicians more than other professional women achieve a healthy balance between fulfillment of their professional and sexual goals. In contrast to the old attitude that womem doctors could only be spinsters and "hen medics," over three-fourths of all women physicians are married (over half, to other physicians), and the majority of them have children.[2] In fact, those physicians who do marry have averaged three children, or slightly more children than reported by other married women in their socio-economic class.[3] According to actual statistics, women entering medicine also have statistically a far greater probability of combining marriage and a career than women beginning graduate work in the physical or social sciences.

Sociologists and psychologists, as well as popular writers, have explored the conflicts or assets (depending on their point of view) which arise when a woman takes on the responsibilities of a career

[1] Lotte Bailyn, "Notes on the role of choice in the psychology of professional women," in Robert J. Lifton (ed.), *The Woman in America* (Boston: Houghton Mifflin, 1965), p. 237.

[2] Lee Powers, Harry Wiesenfelder, and Rexford C. Parmelee, "Practice patterns of women and men physicians," Preliminary Report (October, 1966), Tables 4–B and 7.

[3] "The case against the female M.D." *Medical Economics* (December, 1961).

in addition to her family. The arguments against—neglect of spouse and children, aggressive competition between marital partners, undermining the "bread-winning status" of the man, etc.— have been offset by glowing reports of the positive results: increased stimulation in the home, greater compatibility between husband and wife, and above all, fulfillment of the woman's potential. The most reasonable viewpoint on the subject is probably the one given by Elizabeth Herzog of the Children's Bureau, who states:

> Consensus of the research to date is that gainful employment of the wife is not a significant factor in either marriage success or failure. It is a peg on which conflict can be hung, a socially approved area in which to disagree.[4]

For the woman and those dependent on her love and services, being a physician may imply more than the ordinary amount of energy taken away from the family. While women generally avoid professions such as engineering because of their "masculine" image, Alice Rossi reports that in her sample of college-educated women this was not the problem; rather, "four out of five say that women do not go into medicine because 'it is too demanding to combine with family responsibilities.' "[5] According to Rossi:

> This seems to flow from an image of the doctor modelled on the general practitioner of horse-and-buggy days, on call night and day, seven days a week. There is no room in this image for the contemporary partnerships, group practices, increased specialization, staff appointments, restricted house calls, etc., which are increasingly characteristic of the medical profession. Training to become a doctor may be hard for a woman unless she postpones marriage or at least child-bearing, but once she has a medical degree, a pediatric partnership or appointments as a staff pathologist or

[4] Elizabeth Herzog, *Children of Working Mothers* (Washington: U.S. Department of Health, Education, and Welfare, Children's Bureau, 1960).

[5] Alice S. Rossi, "Why so few women become engineers, doctors, and scientists." In Jacquelyn A. Mattfield and Carol G. Van Aken (eds.), *Women and the Scientific Professions* (Cambridge: The M.I.T. Press, 1965), p. 97.

anesthetist might actually provide more flexibility of routine and shorter hours of work than a job as a laboratory technician.[6]

Rossi's evaluation of the possibilities for relaxed scheduling in the life of a woman physician may be overly optimistic. Most women do not practice part-time, and many give 60 to 70 hours a week to their profession. In a recent survey, 54.5 per cent of the women physicians reported having worked over 2,000 hours in 1964 (full-time), 30.5 per cent less than 2,000 hours (part-time); another 6.1 per cent reported activity but did not specify hours, and only 8.9 per cent said they were not working at all.[7] The percentage of women reporting relatively full-time activity ranged from 86.4 per cent of the single women to 72.6 per cent of the married women with no children to 55.3 per cent of those with one or two children, to 39.3 per cent of those with three or more children.[8]

Two reasons may be given for the fact that such a high percentage of women doctors work full-time, as opposed to women in other fields. In the first place, because of the shortage of physicians and their vital importance to the community, women physicians may have more of a sense of responsibility to fulfill the demands made on their professional services. Particularly for those in private or group practice, it is nearly impossible to keep down the size of the practice as it tends to grow year by year: when a patient is referred to a doctor, it is hard to say no, even if her 40 hours have already been scheduled. The alternative of a salaried position may provide more clear-cut and regular schedules, but even here part-time often implies taking home papers and records or seeing patients "after hours."

In the second place, without resorting to undue generalization, it is clear that the type of woman who enters medicine is usually endowed with more than average energy and motivation and a desire to work to her full capacity. The obstacles of the pre-medical

[6] *Ibid.*
[7] Powers, Wiesenfelder, and Parmelee, "Practice patterns," Table 10.
[8] *Ibid.*, Table 15.

and medical training years discussed in earlier chapters weed out most of those girls with less willfulness and ambition, and those who survive feel strong enough to want both a career and a family.

Most amazing is the fact that such a large proportion of women in medicine do, to a large degree, follow through with their career plans. Whatever the girl's hopes may be, however, it is her husband, if she marries, who ultimately determines the possibility of continuing in her profession while being a wife and mother. Edna Rostow, in an article on "Conflict and Accommodation" in the lives of American women, states:

> For a woman to perform in two worlds, as men do, her marriage must countenance her dual goals and support her in seeking them. The marriage relation is seen more and more consciously as a process in which husband and wife co-operate on many levels in order to permit each separately and both together to achieve a number of goals and satisfy a number of needs—not the least of them the need to control or eliminate destructive elements between them . . . For a woman to accept from her husband the kind of help that man has traditionally taken as his due from his wife, however, can be an emotionally complicated experience for both.[9]

"The right husband" is one of the most common requirements set up by women physicians themselves for combining a medical career with marriage. Without a husband who actively supports his wife's career, most women physicians maintain that there can be only two solutions: divorce, or sacrifice of the medical career. The self-conscious gratitude of these women toward their husbands for helping them maintain their professional lives is impressive. Even those who acknowledge that their husbands give little practical assistance to ease their work burden—"He usually reads the paper or looks over his journal while I do the dishes"—emphasize the importance of their husbands' emotional support. "He tells me

---

[9] Edna G. Rostow, "Conflict and Accommodation," in Robert J. Lifton (ed.), *The Woman in America*, p. 224.

I'm so much more stimulating to be with, now that I've returned to work," said one woman who had retired to become a full-time housewife while her children were young. "My husband has always been very willing to overlook short-order meals or a rug that needed vacuuming so that I could continue my job at the hospital," another remarked.

Since many women physicians still feel the responsibility to fulfill their traditional duties as housewife and mother, there may be a confusion at times as to how much one should ask of one's husband, or allow him to do when he does offer. In many cases, the lack of time may bring about a simple solution: the wife cannot do everything, and someone else must give a hand somewhere. Feeling themselves to be capable and strong, many women physicians, however, do not like to ask. "I try to get home in time to straighten up the house and make a full-course dinner," said a resident who had been married less than a year. "I don't think it's right for him to have to put on a kitchen apron."

Another woman, who had just finished a strenuous year of internship, described how her husband had rushed home from the hospital (he was already a licensed pathologist) to relieve the baby-sitter and change a diaper, and how he had often spent long evenings alone with their two babies while she had to remain at the hospital. "I used to feel so sorry for him!" she recalled. Her experiences during this period had convinced her to take a residency program which would allow her to be home regularly and for long enough periods to hold up her end of the familial responsibilities. Although she made no mention of her husband's having complained, it was obvious that she—and probably both of them—could not adapt to such a reversal of roles for long.

Because many of the responsibilities and roles are not the traditional ones which husband and wife expect when they first marry, compromise and adaptation become a very conscious part of the lives of women physicians and their husbands. Dr. Rosa Lee Nemir, former President of the American Medical Women's Association, described the process of adaptation in her own marriage in the following way:

> There are periods when one or the other ascends, but you have to cherish both lives. It's like putting bulbs in the ground at the right time. You always have to keep your interests and wits alive. When it's a crucial period in my medical life my husband has to become a partner and give me emotional support. Then the next year I may say, I'll pay more attention to you than I ever did before.

When the marriage occurs after the couple's ways of living and working are rather set, the adjustment may take a somewhat different course than when the two are starting out. If both members are far along in their careers when the marriage occurs, they may give each other greater leeway and be less inclined to mold the other in his or her image, since their ways of living and working have already settled into a somewhat rigid form. One woman, who put off marriage until she had completed her residency and passed her specialty boards, reported her anxiety as the wedding approached that her career, which meant so much to her, would be disturbed by her new life. She was used to getting up at five in the morning, for instance, to write reports and work on articles; these were her most creative hours of the day. "I asked my fiance if we might have separate bedrooms when we were married," she smiled, "so that I wouldn't disturb him when I did my work. He thought I was crazy, but agreed—if I felt I needed it. Well, the situation never arose. Once I was married, I found that I didn't want to get up in the morning as I had done before. I still did my writing, but I found other, more convenient times to do it."

Marriages among medical students, interns, and residents, while increasing the possibility of financial and other difficulties, bring the partners together at an age when adaptation is usually easier for both. The relatively new concept of a "partnership" marriage is reflected in the burgeoning number of couples who join their private and professional lives in a more co-operative manner than was the norm several decades ago. One young Harvard graduate expressed this attitude jokingly: "All couples should be incorporated, so that whoever hires one of them has to hire the other."

Over half of all husbands of women physicians are themselves doctors. Women physicians, in fact, appear to gravitate towards mates in their own profession more than do women in other fields. In a study of women professionals in New York State, 58 per cent of the women physicians, in contrast to 50 per cent of the women lawyers, 40 per cent of the women dentists, 17 per cent of the women educational administrators, and none of the women in nursing administration were married to men in their own professions.[10] Unfortunately, no data have been gathered on the number of physician-couples who actually practice together or who do co-operative research. A guess is that an increasing number are doing so, although married medical teams are by no means a new phenomenon. At Stanford, Dr. Emile Holman, the distinguished cardiovascular surgeon, and Dr. Ann Purdy, who established the first cardiac clinic for children in San Francisco, were an outstanding example a generation ago.

Even when the husband is in a different profession, there can be an enormous degree of sharing and co-operation. An illustration of the eager involvement of a lawyer in his physician-wife's career is given by Morton Hunt in *Her Infinite Variety*. The lawyer recalls the early years of his marriage when his wife was still a medical student:

> My practice was growing fast and I could have afforded a nice place, but in order to save her travel time I moved in with her into her little dormitory room. For a year and a half, I'd come back to that little place after a long day in court, take her out for a quick dinner, and then help her study until late at night, or help her relax sometimes by telling her stories about my cases, or hobnobbing with the other med students. I got to be the best midnight scrambled-egg cook on an illegal electric burner that you

[10] Rita L. Stafford, "An analysis of consciously recalled motivating factors and subsequent professional involvement for American women in New York state" (unpublished Ph.D. dissertation, School of Education, New York University, 1967), p. 317.

ever heard of. It was a grind, but I really loved the whole atmosphere—it was almost like being on some kind of wartime mission.

And looking back on his life with his wife-physician, he explains:

There *are* times when I think how much simpler it all was for
my father—he would just come home and take his ease, and let
everybody fuss over him. He was the one who counted, and everything was arranged to suit him. Sometimes I wish it were that
way with me. But then Rosalie and I go out to dinner and I see
people our own age sitting opposite each other but staring around
sideways or looking at their food, and not having anything at all
to say to each other. *We're* still like each other's dates—after
eighteen years. We always find each other interesting, and its
amazing to see how she really looks especially pretty and full of
bounce after she's just pulled off a tricky operation and is still all
excited and pleased by it, even though she's really dead-tired. I
can't be sure how all this would have worked out if I weren't
pretty successful in my own field, but I am. She has great respect
for what I do, and she has even come to court a few times to hear
me. She's very much a woman with me, but once in a while, if
she tries to take over a little too much, I call her "Doctor" very
respectfully, and she gets nettled for a minute, and then laughs
and turns it off.[11]

The threat of competition between two professionals married to
each other may, in many cases, be something which is more feared
than actually experienced. "Competition"—a word which to many
women still has such negative connotations that it can barely be
discussed for longer than it takes to make a complete denial of its
existence in their lives—is often a positive glue and source of
stimulation to professional as well as non-professional couples. In
casual discussion, the word may call up visions of the wife increasing her salary to match her husband's, or refusing to carry out those
wifely duties which might make her subservient in her own and
her husband's eyes. As a constructive force, however, competition
may prompt both parties to read outside their fields, to "keep up
with" their mates, or to work hard for a position that the mate will
be proud of. Not only do more men appear to be able today to take

[11] Morton M. Hunt, *Her Infinite Variety* (New York: Harper and
Row, 1962), pp. 281–82.

independently successful wives than ever before, but women professionals still have a long way to go before they become as openly aggressive and competitive as some people fear they are. Most women doctors, because of children or their own lesser aspirations, limit their professional careers and do not succeed to as high a level as their husbands. In the few cases where they have married below their own professional prestige level,[12] there has been an attempt to preserve the traditional ranking. "At work I head a program and manage my duties the way I think best, but at home my husband is the boss, and I like it that way," stated one physician. Another woman who had married a man with no college degree refused a position as chief of a government service because she would outrank her husband socially and economically. Whether or not she unconsciously married someone with less education than she because it would limit her own achievement is difficult to say. In general, women physicians stress the importance of having a husband who is successful in his own world, whatever he does. If the woman feels that his self-confidence is secure and not at stake in her success, she will have the freedom to go as far as she herself wants.

A common notion is that the competition implicit when both mates have professional status will lead more easily to divorce; this attitude is defended by citing the fact that there is a somewhat higher divorce rate among women physicians than among the general female population.[13] However, the higher rate of divorce is probably due much less to competition than to a laissez faire atti-

[12] Although no statistics are available on the number of women physicians married to nonprofessionals, my impression from interviews with women doctors, corroborated by data on women in other professions, suggests that the nonprofessional husband is a rarity. In Ginzberg's study of women receiving graduate training at Columbia University, for instance, only one-fourth had husbands who did not have at least one graduate degree. See Eli Ginzberg and associates, *Life Styles of Educated Women* (New York: Columbia University Press, 1966), p. 25.

[13] Data on physicians from Powers, Wiesenfelder, and Parmelee, "Practice patterns," Table 3. Data on general population from Paul H. Jacobson, *American Marriage and Divorce* (New York: Rhinehart, 1959), p. 159.

tude which can arise when both partners have busy schedules. Because people have such a fear of open aggression in interpersonal relations, they assume that the tragedy of divorce can only stem from the bloody battles which must surely occur when two people are strong. What is more common is the situation in which the physician, extending her highly-controlled manner into her home, allows both of them to drift further and further away until either a divorce occurs or the marriage continues only in name. In interviews with women doctors, one gains the impression that they are sometimes able to shed their husbands in much the same way that a general loses a horse shot from under him—without forfeiting momentum in their careers. A woman doctor who married in the first year of medical school and divorced several years later, admitted that she had felt nothing throughout the whole divorce proceedings—no one around her had guessed that anything was amiss—and she had not even cried during it. One day about a year later, during her internship, an elder physician scolded her in front of a patient for making a sloppy presentation. At this moment, through the tears of professional humiliation, she was able to feel all the accumulated pain of the other experience.

It would be unfair to leave out the positive side of the higher divorce rate among women physicians and other professional women. Having an economically rewarding as well as emotionally fulfilling career, they need marriage neither as the sole financial nor emotional center for their lives. In many cases, where an untrained woman might feel forced to hang on to a bad situation, a self-sufficient doctor would be free to work out a better life.

Physician-Mothers and Conflicting Commitments

In her own way, the modern professional woman may come closer to the Renaissance ideal of self-fulfillment along many lines than her male contemporaries. Although women doctors do not achieve as many "firsts" in their fields as do the men, they usually express themselves in a wider range of abilities and interests over their lives. For this reason, it is often difficult for themselves and others to evaluate their success. According to the psychologist, David McClelland:

> The phrase "part-time" catches a lot of the essence of the feminine style of life in a very practical sense. Women will be part-time daughters, part-time mothers, part-time wives, part-time cooks, part-time intellectuals, part-time workers. They may spend part of their lives being wholly wives and mothers and another part being wholly intellectuals. But their psychology permits this degree of alternation more easily than for a man who will often blindly follow a single course. A woman's success is less easily visible, by the same token, because it consists of the sum of all these activities rather than the result of a single-minded pursuit of one.[14]

The ranks of women physicians, probably more than any other professional women's group, have furnished models to prove that the effective balance of many different activities is one of the more common miracles to be encountered in the world. They have larger families than do women lawyers or academic women and, at the same time, their record for the amount of time given to their profession is better than that of either of the other groups.[15] In a way which is admirable and sometimes frightening, they show a great capacity to have their cake and eat it too.

Needless to say, combining medicine with raising a family is not an easy task: it requires much energy and planning to do well by husband, children, and profession, and, what is equally important, to see that she herself does not suffer. The paradox is that what may appear in one light as perhaps being a little self-indulgent (i.e., having your cake, etc.) yields the practical result of being

[14] David C. McClelland, "Wanted: a new self-image for women," in Robert J. Lifton (ed.), *The Woman in America,* pp. 187–88.

[15] Stafford, "An analysis of consciously recalled motivating factors and subsequent professional involvement" (pp. 346 and 348) compares women physicians and lawyers by the number of hours per week and per year given to the profession. Jessie Bernard, *Academic Women* (Cleveland: Meridian, 1966), pp. 85–95 gives statistics on career patterns among academic women.

placed in a position in which the woman's own subsequent demands cannot be listened to, least of all by herself. She has to operate with a great degree of responsibility, and with the ever-present reminder that she has no right to neglect any of her jobs for relief—because she herself has taken them on. In effect, she is submerging herself in a tunnel of obligations for ten or twenty years, with little time to come up for air, but with the conviction that this is the most satisfying kind of life that can be had.

The dangers to this course are strain and a loss of touch with herself. One psychiatrist said:

> The demands of psychiatric patients on the one hand and of young children on the other are very exhausting, and I am often fatigued. Though I get through at my office each day at 2:00 P.M., I find there is little time to do anything for *myself*.

Some women physicians report that they simply relinquish any thoughts of taking care of themselves while their children are young. For those who continue working throughout this period, it may seem like an extended internship with two centers of crises: the hospital and the home.

Although women doctors have great resources and energy, their assumption of more and more responsibilities may bring them to a limit where one activity must be sacrificed or curtailed for another. The most usual circumstance effecting this occurs when they have children. The appearance of children may solidify a marriage and may help the woman to maintain her feminine identity while working in a man's world, but her capacity for involvement in her career and husband is more likely to undergo reduction. One important medical staff member was asked which of the three—career, husband, or children—was more likely to be put off a little by a woman doctor when the going got rough. Her answer was brief and decisive: "Well, the children certainly don't suffer." When pressed for the next in line, she was a little more evasive and finally said: "I believe, and I think most women physicians believe, that they have a very real duty to use their medical education and serve the community's health problems." The question was dropped at that, but the intimation of who the third-place candidate might be was clear.

With their wives bustling between patients and children (and often having little time for personal adornment or special attentiveness), it is not surprising that husbands often take a more "conservative" line about having the woman return home during the child-rearing years than the women themselves do. In a study of college graduates:

> . . . although one-half of the women thought it appropriate for a woman to take a part-time job if a child is a pre-schooler, only one-third of the men approved. One-fourth of the men and only 14 per cent of the women thought a full-time job should not be taken until the children were "all grown up."[16]

While the man says that having his wife stay home is for the children's sake, this attitude may actually be triggered by his own sense of being the neglected and forgotten party. Such feelings often depart when the woman learns how to juggle her roles and loses some of her time-consuming anxiety; although with all of these responsibilities, the amount of time that the couple has alone together cannot help but decrease. A woman dermatologist, who lived in the suburbs but practiced in the city, told me that she commuted with her husband each morning and evening: their forty-five minutes together on the train was the only guaranteed time during the day which they had alone, and they put it to good use.

When the doctor leaves her position or practice to give birth to her child, an important question for her to settle is: When should she go back? Some stay at home little more than the time needed for the delivery and are back at work a week later. Others try to spend the first six months with the child. Still others feel that they are needed at home during the child's formative years, until he goes off to pre-school or kindergarten. Women physicians inter-

---

[16] Rossi, "Why so few women become engineers, doctors, and scientists," p. 87.

viewed often reported that they had spent much longer at home with one child than with another; their decision to remain at home or return to work was usually determined either by the feasibility of taking maternity leave or by their own energy. (Many hospitals, for instance, still do not guarantee a job to a physician-mother who leaves for six months to have her child, even though men are given two years' military leave.) Of course, personal convictions about child-rearing also play a significant role.

There is confusion among women doctors—probably as great as among the population as a whole in this epoch—about what the needs of a young child are for his mother and what the responsibilities of a mother are to her child. Living in a sea of half-facts and hypotheses and waiting for the "final" research reports to come in (if they ever do), the woman physician goes ahead and does what she feels she has to do. Comparing afterwards her own children and those of her friends and neighbors, she justifies her decision by her children's successes and blames herself for their failures. "If I had stayed at home when he was little, he might not have that allergy," said one. Another who did remain at home for the first few years wondered whether her return to work could have been accomplished with less heartache if she had never tried to become a full-time mother.

Betty Friedan tells of the response of an orthodox Jewish woman, a doctor's wife and herself a physician, to returning to work after devoting years to her husband and four children.

> An unassertive, quiet woman, she exerted almost unbelievable effort to obtain her license after fifteen years of inactivity. She told me apologetically: "You just can't stop being interested. I tried to make myself, but I couldn't." And she confessed that when she gets a night call, she sneaks out guiltily as if she were meeting a lover.[17]

Women who continue working, or who return to work while their children are still in school, often show great determination to

[17] Betty Friedan, *The Feminine Mystique* (New York: Dell, 1963), p. 340.

see that each child gets sufficient care and stimulation. Although the mothers' days are spent away from home, they emphasize the quality of the interaction with their children rather than mere quantity. Some mother-physicians have said they feel that they are able to give their children more when they are working, because they actively enjoy the time spent with them and are not as distracted as they would be were they at home all day long. One mother, and her husband, had bought a house in the country to which the whole family retired every Friday afternoon for a concentrated weekend. As her children grew older and the stimulation of the city outshone the pleasures of the cottage and family life, she devised alternative activities which would continue to bring the family together regularly. Another said that she carefully scanned the newspaper during her coffee breaks at the hospital to plan a weekly excursion with her children. When the day came, she often found herself with several additional children from the neighborhood, which pleased her, since most of their mothers did not work.

Women physicians, even when relatively satisfied with the job they are doing both at home and at work, confess to having the feeling of being torn between their responsibilities in the two areas. As one woman expressed it, "I can't help resenting a lot of the time I spend away from home. I'd like to be able to share more with my children. But it's probably *my* loss more than theirs. . . " Another put it this way: "I feel as if I'm always apologizing, either to my profession when I have to go home, or to other women who say, 'Oh, I couldn't leave my child.' "

Morton Hunt has observed that, "The woman who works although she does not need the money is a thorn in the flesh of her friends."[18] Women doctors are acutely aware of the hostile reactions which their professional commitment arouses in non-working mothers; they may try to keep it a secret at casual social gatherings in order to prevent the "deep freeze" which sometimes ensues

---

[18] Hunt, *Her Infinite Variety*, p. 271.

when it becomes known. One woman said that she rarely heard direct remarks against her. "More often I hear of them via the grapevine: 'You must be making a pile of money.'"

Early one morning, as a physician and mother of three children was hurrying off to work after having solved a crisis with the housekeeper and gotten her oldest off to school, she was stopped by a woman pushing a stroller. "How do you do," said the other woman. "You're Dr. X, aren't you? I'm Dr. So-and-so from down the street. But I gave up medicine to be a mother to my children." The doctor who told me this story added that during the next years she had become a much better friend of her neighbor than their first meeting might have forecasted. Behind the woman's aggressive introduction lay an unhappiness at having given up her profession. (She had dropped out before receiving her license and could find nothing on a part-time basis which she felt would justify the sacrifice of time spent with her children.) After many long talks with the practicing physician, she began studying to pass her boards and eventually found a job which required her service only part of the day, a few days a week; in this manner she slowly returned to medicine. The assistance and encouragement given by the practicing doctor was not merely altruistic, however; as she herself intimated, women who "sacrifice" themselves to family life and raising children always make a professional woman feel a little guilty about maintaining her independent identity.

The Practical Problems of Child Care

One variable in a woman's decision either to continue working or to give up her profession while her children are small is the actual physical help available to her. In much of the writing about women in medicine and how they do or do not fulfill their responsibilities to the profession, the emphasis is placed on inherent motivation—their ability to stick it out no matter what the obstacles—and little attention is given to the very real difficulties they face and what might be done to make it easier for the professional woman with children.

The business of employing a woman to take care of one's children involves many potential obstacles. One of the first considerations is the character of the baby-sitter. Many women physicians, probably because of their original concern for health and their desire to ensure adequate protection in this area, hire retired nurses or nurses' aids to take care of their children. In several instances, the physicians said they had paid a nurse the equivalent of her hospital salary so that she would give up her job to take care of the children. On the other hand, some women felt that in choosing a mother-substitute for the baby, "anyone who is warm and kind" would be satisfactory. One doctor said that she wanted "someone who will tell me when she is disgusted with my children as well as when she thinks they're adorable and has had a good day with them."

The difficulties inherent in even the best mother-substitutes are well known. No other person can feel exactly the same as the mother does about all aspects of child-rearing, and not the worst of eventualities is the mother's suspicion that her child is giving a little too much affection to his baby-sitter. One physician was resentful that her housekeeper had won her little daughter over by a lack of discipline. The woman fed the little girl, instead of forcing her to feed herself—it was less work and quicker, since the housekeeper avoided having to clean up the mess—and then when the mother came home and tried to get the girl to eat her evening meal, the child became quite passive, waiting for her mother to help her the way the other woman did. Another physician commented a little wistfully that her two children ran into the arms of the baby-sitter when the woman arrived each morning, and were often busy with their play when she herself came home.

A physician practicing in the suburbs believed that not enough consideration is given to the "social situation currently facing women who plan to enter careers." Elaborating on her feelings in this respect, she said:

> It is now no longer possible for a woman who has normal desires
> for a family to combine motherhood and a career, largely due to

the increasing impossibility of securing adequate domestic help.
I was able to do it, with some difficulty, when my children were
small and can continue now only because they are old enough
to manage and help out. I would *not* encourage my own daughter
to hope for a career involving commitments outside the home and
then face the frustration of being unable to use her skills and
potential. As a psychiatrist, I am frequently called on to treat the
consequences of this frustration.

I believe that unless the government takes steps to remedy the
present situation, and to free the manpower inherent in married
women, it will only worsen. A career and children today demand
superhuman motivation from a mother which can only include
neglect of children.

Since 1940, resources for child care and household help have
shrunk from 18 per cent of the employed women to 8 per cent; at
the same time, more and more mothers have entered the labor
market.[19] Nothing has been done to raise the status of housekeepers in the United States, and as a result, fewer and fewer women
are willing to offer this service. The decrease is also not surprising
when one considers that the job has few of the protections and
benefits other workers take for granted, and no future or possibility
for advancement. It is at present nearly impossible to find child-
care facilities of sufficient quality to give a working mother the
tranquility needed to do her job well. A general practitioner, who
had obviously had a series of bad experiences, expressed her feelings on the situation rather bluntly:

> No one but derelicts, failures, drifters and convicts even applies.
> To stay with one family more than a month is unusual, and if
> the lady of the house isn't there to supervise, the idea is to steal
> as much as possible either directly or indirectly. No one ever
> heard of training for such a job and the employment agencies are
> interested only in their percentages.

While it is still possible to find good help, it is generally recog-

[19] Margaret Mead and Frances Balgley Kaplan (eds.), *American
Women: Report of the President's Commission on the Status of Women*,
and other publications of the Commission (New York: Charles Scribner's
Sons, 1965), p. 41.

nized that provisions are inadequate. One resident, at the end of her wits, told me that she had had six housekeepers in the past year, all of whom had left unexpectedly, and that she was going to relinquish her position at the end of the month to give her children a more settled life. Another physician said that after many unsuccessful trials, she had finally come upon a way of handling her child-care problems: she hired several women on a part-time basis, often mothers who had themselves children to care for and could thus appreciate the difficulties of a mother with more than one responsibility. With the resources of two or three women at hand, she could nearly always find one of them to cover for her —one of the greatest difficulties of the woman physician who is subject to emergency calls.

Two proposals have recently been made to raise the status of women offering housekeeping and child-care services, thus ensuring a higher quality and greater number of women taking on these jobs. The President's Commission on the Status of Women suggested in its 1963 report that household workers should be unionized, and that facilities should be established to train women in child care.[20]

The women physicians who are at present most contented with their arrangements are probably those with relatives or friends nearby upon whom they can depend. Even the mother-in-law whose child-rearing philosophy seems "outdated," or who is more permissive than one would like her to be, is more apt to be a loving and dependable baby-sitter than a stranger. In addition, it is a rare relative who demands the same salary as a woman hired on the outside, and the saving of this expense can be a great boon to the mother who wants to work, but who, under normal conditions, would not have been able to finance it.

Three alternatives are open to the physician-mother determined to work but unable to secure adequate housekeeping or child care in her own locality. The first, the importing of domestic help from

[20] *Ibid.*, pp. 40 and 224.

Europe, has become more widespread in recent years. The young women secured in this way provide the family with the stimulation of a foreign language and tradition. They also bring their problems of adjusting to a new, bewildering society, which gives the employer an added responsibility that may be enriching or troublesome, depending on the situation. The total cost of hiring a foreign girl is usually no more than domestic help.

The second alternative is the day-care center. Although such institutions are still rare, government-run centers have been established in most of the metropolitan areas of the United States, and many large hospitals now have crèches and nurseries for their personnel. The reluctance of women physicians to use these centers is based perhaps on an emotional connection with the Brave New World picture of depersonalized child care. And there is an association with the lower-classes, since many centers are presently in lower-class housing projects and/or connected to welfare centers. A resident at a city hospital observed that while there was a crèche in the hospital for the children of employees, it had become exclusively the place for the children of janitorial help, aids, and perhaps a minority of nurses. Few of the physicians in the hospital had heard of its existence, and still fewer would consider leaving their children there, even though doing so would give them the opportunity to drop in and see the child during the day. A hospital administrator said that when a crèche in his hospital had first opened, he had encouraged women doctors and other higher-status personnel to use it, but they had taken the conservative position of waiting to see how it would turn out first. In the interim the crèche had become utilized by unskilled and semi-skilled personnel. "They should have come in right at the beginning, to set the pace!" he said.

Interestingly, even in the U.S.S.R. and other Eastern European socialist countries where women are actively encouraged to work, the official attitudes towards child-care facilities have not been completely ironed out. The majority of working women in Russia have no choice but to use domestic help or to raise the children themselves, and, as a result, they end up bearing a disproportionate share of the work load. Government policy itself has appeared to favor this solution.

> Although the government has allocated substantial investment funds over the years to the expansion of child-care facilities, it has been unwilling to assign this program sufficient resources to satisfy demand. On the contrary, it has chosen to compel most working women to make their own arrangements—with members of their families or outside help—for the care of their young children. This policy can hardly be considered beneficial to the working mothers. From the standpoint of the regime's overriding goal of economic growth, however, the imposition of hardship on the working mother and a slightly lower rate of participation of women in the labor force have apparently been considered preferable to the diversion of investment funds and other resources to additional child-care facilities.[21]

At a panel discussion in Prague on love, sex, and the family in January, 1967, Milan Novak, a repairman and poet, spoke against women who turn their children over to "cold and uninterested institutions." Mr. Novak demanded that the state pay mothers a living wage for the job of raising children. "Raising children is a form of production, too," he said, "and a Socialist state owes wages according to productivity."[22]

While this idea may sound far-fetched, the President's Commission on the Status of Women argued for something quite similar, realizing that it could not be an immediate solution. The report stated, "The idea of treating homemaking as having a real monetary value, and so a kind of dignity, has important repercussions for women's choices of where and how they'll work, for it could do much to change the present status of the woman domestic worker."[23]

A third solution—along with foreign maids and day-care centers—is for the doctor to practice in an office in her own home. While some assistance with cleaning and even child care may still be

[21] Norton Dodge, *Women in the Soviet Economy* (Baltimore: The Johns Hopkins Press, 1966), p. 241.

[22] "Sex advice given by Czech panel," *New York Times* (January 19, 1967).

[23] Mead and Kaplan, *American Women*, p. 187.

needed, she is nearby to supervise and to help in case an emergency should arise. By staying at home, she can cut down on the extra costs of working outside: transportation, lunches, etc. Practicing at home also provides a kind of relaxation which is impossible with any outside job. Those who have adopted it to their satisfaction are often the most zealous partisans for this approach. Dr. Joanne Denko, a psychiatrist, reports in the *Journal of the American Medical Women's Association* that, having set up an office on an enclosed porch of her home, she is free to treat child patients on this porch or in her back yard at the sandbox. She can schedule her patients to coincide with her young son's nap-time, or in the evening when his father is home to take care of him. By making use of this flexible scheduling, she is able to control her own son's upbringing far more than she could if she were away at the office during the daytime. "In these years before he goes to school I try to teach him things he won't learn there. I make a conscious effort to impress on him values I consider important, rudiments of scientific method, and sensitivity to beauty."[24] She lists a series of such educational experiences: introducing him to forms, colors, smells, and textures in nature, encouraging him to have scientific observation but "not to discourage in him the imaginative, metaphoric, almost poetic way children think until adults stifle it," and going for long walks in the country.

> All these pursuits are inordinately time-consuming and would not be possible if I were either a full-time physician or a standard harassed wife-housekeeper-cook-nurse-mother. Admittedly, the investment by society in my education is not now bringing maximal returns. But this is my compromise with the investment I make in my child.[25]

This points up one of the problematic characteristics of working at home: that it is more suitable to part-time than full-time work, and those who begin it with plans for the latter schedule usually switch to the former. Even doctors who continue full-time work

[24] Joanne D. Denko, "Managing a practice and a home simultaneously; one woman's solution," *J. Amer. Med. Wom. Ass.* 20, no. 8 (1965):765.
[25] *Ibid.*

feel a loss of the demarkation between their family and professional lives. A pediatrician who had maintained an office in her house for a time while her children were young observed that, in retrospect, she thought the quality of her work had not been as good as it would have been had she found someone to assume entire responsibility for the children while she went to an office. An additional problem (although one which can be overcome) is that contact with other doctors—and thus referrals—decrease; for the woman who goes immediately from training into such a practice, it can take some time to build up a remunerative clientele.

*   *   *   *

A universal complaint among women physicians, whether they employ full-time housekeepers or share the job with part-time workers, is the cost of help to substitute for them at home. Many pay up to $100 a week for full-time help, and the fees may actually be higher when the household helper lives in. During the internship and residency, if the doctor has children, her salary may easily be less than what she pays her housekeeper or baby-sitter. If she is in a part-time program, she may spend double her salary from the hospital for someone to take care of her children. The Radcliffe Institute is the only organization until now to realize the importance of this cost in discouraging the mother from continuing her career: Radcliffe physicians-in-training receive the difference between salary and child-care expenses, so that they will not sustain a heavy financial loss through training.

Even with a full salary, many women physicians do not add substantially to their family's total income while the children are young. Some resign themselves to not earning this additional income, but their husbands may be less reconciled, particularly if they are concerned about the welfare of the children with a working mother and wonder what is gained by the wife's job. According to a *New York Times* article on the subject:

> The $15,000-a-year wife married to a husband who earns $20,000 adds about $3,300 to the family's net income, after taxes and her expenses of $5,000 for a housekeeper or nurse for her two children and $1,500 for her own lunches, extra clothes, carfare, and

the like. The family has about $3,300 a year more because she works than if they depended on the husband's income alone. In the case of lower salary levels the advantage is much less.[26]

Two solutions might be offered to this problem: government subsidy for child-care expenses, or tax deductions for the cost of housekeeping and baby-sitting to the working mother. The latter approach is more widely known and espoused by women doctors. It has a plausible justification: a man can deduct his business expenses, while a woman cannot take off the child-care salary she pays, although it is an expense necessary for her work. A baby-sitter is considered a cost which must be borne by the woman alone; the government wants women to work, but thus far has provided no encouragement.

> How my blood used to boil as I would drive to the hospital in my business-expense-deducted automobile after paying $10.00 in cash for the middle-of-the-night babysitter without whom I could not practice medicine. No deduction. But as for the car, well I could always walk . . .

Such problems are not unique to women physicians. At the Governor's Conference on Women in New York in the fall of 1966, working women of all professions reported that their salaries could barely meet the costs of their going to work, and the request was made that child-care expenses be tax deductible. At present, deductions for child care extend only to those women whose incomes are necessary for the support of the family: in other words, those who are divorced, widowed, or for some other reason the sole support, or those whose income combined with their husband's does not exceed the minimum level of $6,000. While it is true that mother-physicians may have to make more concessions than they are presently willing to make—accepting crèches and day-care centers, for example—the government also has a responsibility to ease the burden of these women if their skills and knowledge are to be fully utilized.

[26] Elizabeth Fowler, "Personal finance; working wife finds that her pay doesn't double the family's income," *New York Times* (December 29, 1966).

X

THE PRACTICING WOMAN PHYSICIAN

The Needs in Medicine, and the
Contributions of Women Physicians

The preceding chapters have concentrated to a large extent on what goes into the training and life of a woman physician. Little attention has been given as yet to one of the most pressing questions: should more women be encouraged to enter medicine? The notion that training a woman in medicine is a luxury rather than a valuable investment, and that each increment of her advanced training is one more extravagance rather than the chance for further contribution, must be refuted if the answer is to be yes. Training more women doctors must be shown to be a worthwhile venture from the point of view not only of the women themselves but of society.

In the past few years, the debate has gone back and forth as to what constitutes an adequate medical supply in this country. The ratio of physicians to the population has dropped during the twentieth century: one source reports that while "In 1902, we had one doctor for every 568 patients, in 1960, we had one for every 709."[1] In addition, the average citizen today appears to consult a doctor twice as often as he did in 1930.[2] Obviously, the administration of medicine has also changed, so that in treating some cases a physician may be able to work more efficiently, while in others—surgery is the most often cited—increased knowledge may result in the practice of medicine consuming more time. The designation of traditional but routine duties to para-medical personnel (delivery of

[1] David Rutstein, M.D., "Do you really want a family doctor?" *Harper's Magazine* (October, 1960), p. 145.

[2] Selig Greenberg, "The decline of the healing art," *Harper's Magazine* (October, 1960), p. 133.

babies, immunization, history-taking) may contribute to the greater efficiency of doctors in the future. However, new governmental programs such as Medicare or Medicaid may also increase the need for physicians' services, although to what extent has not yet been determined. Eli Ginzberg, in an article questioning the physician shortage, suggests that the greatest impact of these governmental programs may be in the demand for additional nursing services.[3]

The tremendous growth of medical technology has also changed the geographical distribution of physicians: whereas doctors used to be spread rather evenly over the United States, covering urban, suburban, and rural areas alike, elaborate and costly machinery requiring highly specialized knowledge now holds the newly-trained physician in urban centers, where he can practice the modern brand of medicine which he has been taught. Increased knowledge has also changed the nature of the individual specialties, shifting the responsibilities from one to another and creating greater or lesser needs for physicians in the various fields.

All this is only to say that "the shortage of medical personnel" is not a simple fact. While some experts believe that a 30 per cent increase in the number of physicians now graduating annually must be trained by 1975 if adequate medical service is to be available, others maintain that there is no physician shortage,[4] or that only a more equitable distribution of physicians both geographically and among the various specialties can lead to good health service throughout the country.[5] In support of the latter opinion, it has been pointed out that in Israel, where one physician serves only 416 people, there is complaint of a "physician shortage," while Sweden, with only one physician for every 1,000 of the

[3] Eli Ginzberg, "Physician shortage reconsidered," *New Eng. J. Med.* 275, no. 2 (1966):85.

[4] *Ibid.*

[5] *The Crisis in Medical Services and Medical Education*, report on an exploratory conference, Ft. Lauderdale, Florida, sponsored by the Commonwealth Fund and Carnegie Corporation of New York (February, 1966).

population, boasts one of the highest health standards in the world.[6]

Until now, one of the most common arguments against training women doctors has gone something like: "With such a shortage of physicians, we have to get the optimum amount of service out of every one we train. We can't possibly waste precious medical school space on someone who may not practice temporarily, or who may only practice part-time." Obviously, unless it were ascertained that there were a numerical superfluity of physicians—a highly unlikely eventuality!—it would be difficult to ask medical schools to make it a policy to accept far larger proportions of women solely on the basis of the amount of time they may subsequently give to their professions. A comparison of the practice patterns of men and women physicians graduating between 1931 and 1956 showed that almost 9 per cent of the women were inactive, in contrast to less than 1 per cent of the men. In addition, only 54.5 per cent of the women worked full time, while 88.8 per cent of the men had full-time practices.[7] Although many women, particularly if not married, devote 60–80 hours a week to their profession, women physicians on the whole do not put in the same long schedules as men.[8] Nor do they see as many patients per hour as the men do, since they generally spend a longer time with each one.[9] However, as an editorial in the *New England Journal of Medicine* said on the goal of eliminating all the "slack" from a physician's time, "it is perhaps even more important that the milk of human kindness not be squeezed out . . ."[10]

If physicians are merely machines whose value is judged by the

[6] Statistics from the *Statistical Abstract of Sweden* (1966), and *Israeli Government Year Book* (1966).

[7] Lee Powers, Harry Wiesenfelder, and Rexford C. Parmelee, "Practice patterns of women and men physicians," Preliminary Report (October, 1966), Table 1.

[8] *Ibid.*, Tables 9–11.

[9] *Ibid.*, Table 18.

[10] "The physician shortage," *New Eng. J. Med.* 275, no. 2 (1966):110.

quantity of cases they can deal with in a given period of time, women would not necessarily be more encouraged to enter medicine. If it is found that physicians must be able to be moved from one location to another according to regional need, women may again be found slightly less useful as physicians than men, since they are traditionally dependent on the location of their husbands. But it is questionable whether male physicians will submit to being moved from place to place either. In any case, future physicians will probably not be redistributed throughout rural areas to any great extent, but transportation sources will have to bring patients to urban centers. Since women doctors have consistently accepted salaried positions more willingly than men, the increasing demand for physicians in hospitals, clinics, and health centers should work in favor of admitting more women into medicine, as should the fact that they enter specialties of increasingly acute need, such as pediatrics, psychiatry, and public health.

What probably does and should above all justify a free and open attitude towards women in medicine is the large number of contributions which they have made in research, teaching, public service, and private practice. In some cases they have made these contributions because, as women, they have had their own specific perception of needs; in other instances, their intelligence, training, and determination to work out a problem or to devote themselves to a given area of service has been indistinguishable from a man's best work. It is true that—as with any field where creativity is demanded—individuals of another sex, race, or ethnic group are valuable in opening up new areas of investigation. In medicine, women have been noted for their pioneering work in child psychiatry, congenital deformities, cancer research, and a wide range of problems related to public health.

The work of women physicians in family planning demonstrates the impressive contribution which a group can make because of its own particular concerns. In 1914 Margaret Sanger, a public health nurse, published 100,000 copies of a pamphlet called, "Family Limitation,"[11] and two years later—after fleeing to Europe to avoid jail—came back to open the first birth control clinic in the United States in the Brownsville section of Brooklyn. Women physicians in New York kept the clinic open while Margaret Sanger served a term in jail in 1916. When the Clinical Research Bureau opened as an adjunct to the clinic in 1923, Dr. Hannah Stone became its supervising doctor, sacrificing her hospital affiliation by accepting the position. It was 1937 before the American Medical Association came out in support of birth control, and many years later before discussions of methods were considered a fit topic for scientific meetings. The Margaret Sanger Research Bureau is still staffed largely by women physicians who see 15,000 patients a year, offering contraceptive and fertility services, Papanicolaou tests, and premarital advice. Training is also given to physicians, medical students, nurses, and other professionals.

The American Medical Women's Association has consistently taken progressive stands relating to the health and welfare of women. Having stood at the forefront of family planning in the years when the battle was being fought, the AMWA is one of the few medical organizations to take a position in favor of liberalization of the abortion laws. Many individual women doctors all over the United States are also working privately toward abortion reform. One physician who had spent much of her time lobbying in the state capitol said, "I think this is a number one problem for women, if only because of the high death rate due to the way the system now works. And I also think it should be a number one concern for women doctors."

The Memorial Sloan-Kettering Cancer Center represents another organization in which women have played an active role. One of the few women department chairman in the country, Dr. M. Lois Murphy, heads the Department of Pediatrics at the center's clinical unit, Memorial Hospital for Cancer and Allied Diseases. Some of

[11] Diana L. Shaman, "Margaret Sanger: the mother of birth control," in *Coronet* (March, 1966).

the women doctors at the center work primarily in the laboratory, while still others are concerned with the actual treatment of the patient with cancer. Dr. Marguerite Sykes, for instance, is a practicing internist who has for many years published her research in chemotherapy, particularly relating to cancers of the endometrium and skin cancer. Dr. Alice Moore is exclusively engaged in laboratory research. Recently she has concentrated on studies of lymphocytes, an area which has come into increasing focus in the treatment of cancer and other diseases. Drs. Florence Chu and Ruth Snyder approach the treatment of cancer through their training in radiation. Several women, among them Dr. Elizabeth Pickett, are surgeons. The field of cancer research is a particularly germinal one, which is constantly growing as research on cells extends to studies of virology, immunology, and heredity. Because of its stimulation as well as its tremendous pertinence, many women are attracted to the field, and often they come to it through the specialties in which large numbers of women are regularly trained—pediatrics, internal medicine, obstetrics-gynecology, pathology, and radiology.

*   *   *   *

Dr. Florence Sabin is an example of a great medical woman scientist who did significant research in several areas, and whose life clouds some of the distinctions between feminine and masculine contributions to medicine. She was born in 1871 in Central City, Colorado, the second daughter of a miner father and housewife mother.[12] When Florence was seven, her mother died in childbirth, and she and her sister Mary were sent to a series of schools and relatives who gave them "second homes." She graduated from Smith College in 1893 and spent the next three years teaching in order to save money for her medical education.

In 1896, Florence Sabin entered The Johns Hopkins Medical School. An important inspiration to her plans for a medical career

---

[12] The following account of Dr. Sabin's life is taken from Elinor Bluemel, *Florence Sabin: Colorado Woman of the Century* (Boulder, Colo.: University of Colorado Press, 1959).

had been Dr. Ann Preston, then Dean of the Woman's College of Pennsylvania. At Hopkins, Florence Sabin came under the tutelage of Dr. Franklin Mall in the Anatomy Department and, before graduating, received several awards for independent studies of the lymphatic vessels, which Dr. Mall had encouraged her to conduct. While still in medical school, she also made a three-dimensional model of the medulla, pons, and mid-brain, which was to remain the classic teaching-aid in medical schools for many years. Her success in these areas of pure research encouraged her to devote her training to laboratory work, although few women before her had entered the research side of medicine.

During the next years, first as a Fellow and then an Assistant in the Department of Anatomy at Johns Hopkins, Florence Sabin continued to work under Dr. Mall. In her characteristic way of adopting other families, she also became close friends with the entire Mall household. When Dr. Mall died in 1917, she wrote his biography, which was a sensitive analysis of Mall's intellectual and scientific growth and also an account of Johns Hopkins during the years he was there.

Dr. Mall's death put Florence Sabin next in line for promotion to full professor in the Department of Anatomy. When she was overlooked for the position—probably because she was a woman— her students rebelled, and some even thought she should leave Johns Hopkins. In the end, she was made Professor of Histology, since there was a vacancy in that department. Her failure to receive the professorship in Anatomy did not discourage her, although she did feel differently towards Johns Hopkins after that. As her biographer remarks: ". . . she was disappointed, not only for herself, but for all the women in medicine. She felt that she had failed both herself and them."[13]

Dr. Sabin proceeded from the study of the lymph system to that of the origin of blood vessels, which led her to questions about the reaction of body cells to tuberculosis, and to some important dis-

[13] *Ibid.*, p. 87.

coveries about that illness. In 1924, she was awarded membership in the National Academy of Science—the first woman to be given this acclamation. Her work attracted the attention of Dr. Simon Flexner—one of the three illustrious Flexner brothers—who was Director of the Rockefeller Institute for Medical Research. In 1925 he asked her to join his staff and to set up a Department of Cellular Studies for work on problems in immunity.

Florence Sabin's years at the Rockefeller Institute constitute the second stage of her professional life. Her position as full-time researcher left her no opportunity to teach, a job which she had loved and done well. She now became involved in intensive studies of blood as related to tuberculosis, and the biological properties and significance of the various chemical fractions which went into the cause and mechanism of infection. For the first time, under her department, an inter-institutional research program was coordinated for the advancement of knowledge about tuberculosis: although this group did not find a cure for the illness, their work led to a fruitful study of other blood diseases. When Dr. Sabin resigned from the Rockefeller Institute at the age of 67, she had published 40 scientific articles in her own name and 74 in collaboration with her colleagues at Johns Hopkins and the Rockefeller Institute. Not only had she been prolific in her publications, but her work had been consistently of the highest quality.

Now began what were supposed to have been her retirement years. Florence Sabin returned to Colorado to join her sister Mary, a retired school teacher. But Dr. Sabin's own temperament made her retirement impossible. After several years of involving herself in a multitude of short-term issues without any specific direction, she entered public life again, and in 1944 was appointed Chairman of the Subcommittee on Health in the state of Colorado. During the next decade she worked under four governors, traveling back and forth across the state to interest voters in issues of public health and preventive medicine; for the first time, she found herself giving speeches to large crowds of laymen, milkmen's associations, and medical societies. She vigorously investigated sewage systems, dairy farms, psychiatric and tuberculosis sanitoriums. In

1947 during the administration of Governor Knous, the Sabin Health Bills, were passed—eventually lowering the death rate in Colorado from one of the highest in the country to one of the lowest. The all-encompassing level of her concern with unsanitary conditions is indicated by the bill she sponsored which outlawed public bubble fountains, because she considered them germ receptacles. Such concern for mundane details, and even the ability to see them, has been a characteristic feature of women's contributions to public health. In 1948, she was appointed Manager of Health and Charity for Denver. Five years later she died in her home at the age of 82.

Florence Sabin's life is relevant not only because of what she contributed to the world, but also because it represents a pattern of life for the unmarried physician. In the case of Dr. Sabin, she felt that she was too unattractive to get married. But contrary to having a lonely or empty life, she was able to fill it with more than her share of deeply satisfying friendships. She was not one of the independent feminists who existed in large numbers at the time; and, in fact, for a good part of her career, she seemed to need to work under a man whom she felt had superior intelligence and to devote her labors to him. This was true not only of her relationship with Dr. Mall, but also with Dr. Flexner and his two brothers. One of her closest friendships was with Ned Sheldon the playwright, who became blind at the age of 37. Through him she kept up an interest in literature and the theatre, reading to him when she had the time, and attending theatrical productions to tell him what they were like.

As a teacher, she was said to have treated her students with maternal concern, setting up strict problems which stretched their intellectual capacities, but always searching to find out what they wanted to know and not forcing her own attitudes on them. No doubt she channeled some of her mother-instincts into teaching, as well as into the children of her many friends and acquaintances. She was fond of buying them children's books, and always read the book carefully before she presented it.

In Florence Sabin's generation, it was common for an intellec-

tual woman not to marry. The men in the medical schools no
longer thought of their women colleagues as potential wives after
these women had lasted out their first year. Sir William Osler had
said, "There are three classes of human beings: men, women, and
women physicians," which gives us some idea of their early reception in the medical world.

Another example of a single woman of that generation who ex-
celled in medicine is Dr. Connie Guion: at the age of 86 she continues her phenomenal work in internal medicine at Cornell University Medical College, after a long history of achievement. It
was she who founded the Comprehensive Care Program, extending the personal all-around attention of the general practitioner
into the large city clinics. The program, which coordinates all
aspects of medical care for each patient, has affected hospitals
throughout the United States and other countries as well.

There is no doubt that it is easier for a woman who is unmarried
to give herself completely to medicine and to make the kind of top-
level contributions which the best men have made. Similarly, it is
clear that so-called "spinster doctors" can lead fulfilling lives outside of the laboratory or clinic.

These adamant comments of one questionnaire respondent, who
received an M.D. in 1932 and who has been married for thirty
years but has had no children, are rather interesting in that they
deal directly with this issue. She believes that a good marriage and
a full medical career are almost impossible, and goes on to say:

> The modern quest for fulfillment seems crazy to me. To be busy,
> useful, needed, good at what you do and able to take personal
> pride in your accomplishments is what makes a person happy and
> satisfied. Sex and matrimony have little bearing on it. Spinsters,
> grandmothers, childless career women all build good satisfying
> lives when they have within themselves zest for living, curiosity
> about this whole world, enthusiastic interest in people and things
> around them, and throw themselves wholeheartedly into living
> as best they know how. They are happy and satisfied. You forget
> that few persons, doctors included, have everything as they
> dreamed it. You take second best here, turn this bit of tragedy
> into something good, and turn to other things when a facet of life

goes sour. From childhood on we adjust and adjust, to wars, and crimes, and difficult personalities, and personal tragedies and disappointments. "Fulfillment" and happiness are by-products of living, nothing you can capture by a program of questing.

Although an increasing proportion of women doctors do feel they are entitled to the satisfactions of both a career and a family, it is still generally true that the addition of marriage and children tends to lower professional achievement. In Dykman and Stalnaker's "Survey of Women Physicians Graduating from Medical School, 1925–40,"[14] single women doctors stood between married women, on the one hand, and men physicians, on the other, in their degree of involvement and level of achievement in the medical world. In comparison to their married women colleagues, they had held more hospital appointments, published more articles and books, were more often members of medical societies and participated more actively in them. In the case of publication of books and membership in honorary societies, in fact, single women exceeded

TABLE 10–1. DISTRIBUTION OF FULL-TIME AND PART-TIME PROFESSIONAL ACTIVITY IN 1964 FOR WOMEN BY MARITAL STATUS AND NUMBER OF CHILDREN

Marital status, number of children, 1964		Full-time + 2,000 hrs.	Part-time − 2,000 hrs.	No activity	Total
Single	No.	244	32	8	284
	(*per cent*)	86.0	11.2	2.8	100
Married, no children	No.	58	23	7	88
	(*per cent*)	65.8	26.2	8.0	100
Married, 1–2 children	No.	153	135	20	308
	(*per cent*)	49.6	43.9	6.5	100
Married, 3 + children	No.	161	177	72	410
	(*per cent*)	39.3	43.1	17.6	100

Source: Lee Powers, Harry Wiesenfelder, and Rexford C. Parmelee, "Practice patterns of women and men physicians," Preliminary Report (October, 1966), Table 16.

[14] Roscoe A. Dykman and John M. Stalnaker, "Survey of women physicians graduating from medical school, 1925–40," *J. Med. Educ.* 32, no. 3 (March, 1957):28–29.

the men. An updating of this study by Powers *et al.* in 1966 showed that the number of hours given to the medical profession is directly related to the size of the family which the woman has to deal with in addition to her medical responsibilities.

Some of the reasons for curtailed activity due to children have been given in the preceding chapter. Time may be the predominant element limiting mother-physicians in their practice and their participation in medical groups and societies. But for some of these women, the expense of increased involvement is another important determent: in addition to baby-sitting costs, there are fees to the medical groups and malpractice insurance costs necessary for practicing. None of these fees runs on a graded scale, so that a woman wanting to have a somewhat less demanding practice is forced to pay the same high fees as those receiving an income from a large practice.

It has been noted that there is a higher turnover rate among women in part-time salaried positions than among those in full-time work or among men in part-time positions.[15] This turnover may be largely due to the difficulty of justifying the expense of part-time work when the remuneration is so low.

The siphoning of imagination and energy into domestic areas during the woman's particularly creative years has been given as a reason for the fewer publications among women with children than those who are single or childless. Although this may be a factor, innumerable scientific articles have been written by women with children. Many women doctors who do conduct extensive research while raising their families are involved in an area such as pediatrics or child psychiatry, which can be nourished by their experiences at home.

One such woman whom I interviewed—Dr. Ruth Lawrence—had the distinction of being the mother of eight children as well as an Associate Professor in Pediatrics at the University of Rochester.

---

[15] John Kosa and Robert E. Cocker, "The female physician in public health; conflict and reconciliation of the sex and professional roles," *Sociology and Social Research* 49, no. 3 (April, 1965):296–97.

She has worked in the past on a program to improve the health of children in the Rochester public schools, and more recently, has conducted a follow-up study on women graduates of the University of Rochester Medical School. Her teaching duties are listed as part-time, although Dr. Lawrence remarked that "the only thing part-time about the job is the salary." When a colleague left for another part of the country, she inherited the additional chore of directing a toxic-care center for children who have just swallowed poison: her home telephone number is the same as that of the Center, so that she can be reached easily in an emergency.

Not surprisingly, Dr. Lawrence saw that the most important skill for a woman doctor with a family is learning to use time efficiently. She felt that it was entirely possible for a person to do the same job in a so-called "part-time" position as a full-time one if the dawdling and socializing were cut out. "I read my mail and drink my cup of coffee at home, not on clinic time." She confessed with pleasure that there were a few colleagues on the staff who had never found out that she was only part-time. "I've never lied about it; but if someone comes up to me and asks me to do something at four in the afternoon I don't say, 'I have to run home and take care of my kids'; I say, 'Let's see, how about fitting it in Wednesday at 10:30?' It works much better that way and there's less resentment all around. I don't go around with a big sign saying, 'Part-time'!"

When she reaches home around 3 p.m., Dr. Lawrence relieves her domestic help and sits down to complete her reports. She subscribes to a taped digest of medical research, and listens to it while ironing or sewing—a method she strongly recommends to other women doctors for keeping up to date. She and her husband, an anesthesiologist, make just enough money to meet their high expenses with eight children, but they feel that they went into medicine because they loved it, not as a way of getting rich. As Dr. Lawrence says, "When I'm running downstairs with my fifth load of wash Saturday morning, I think about a good lecture I've just given or maybe even a child's life I've saved, and it kind of gives you a nice feeling."

The pleasant feeling of having accomplished something worthwhile, and the sense of being on the right side of the ledger with the world in all relations, are strong, necessary inducements for many women in the daily practice of medicine. These rewards reflect a desire for moral uprightness on the part of the typical hardworking doctor, which may at times have overtones of self-righteousness, but which also drives him or her to make large personal sacrifices for the community.

The Reception of Women Doctors

One of the main topics of concern to women physicians is their reception by the general public, since their own ease in practicing is to a large extent dependent on their patients' willingness to accept them as physicians. No surveys have been conducted on the degree of preference for women doctors since the 1940's, when Josephine Williams and her associates interviewed middle-class women in the Chicago area. By asking them to shuffle a series of cards on which were printed various classifications of doctors, she found that:

> . . . the women physicians' status among these middle-class urban women patients is comparable to the male physician's status among persons of a different faith. An experienced woman is preferred to a very young male doctor and to an experienced male Negro doctor.[16]

While the number of women in medicine has increased in the last twenty-five years since this survey was taken, it is likely that a similar rank order would be found today.

Interestingly, the Negro woman, who might appear to have two strikes against her—sex and race—finds no lack of opportunity to use her training. A Negro doctor, who graduated from Woman's Medical College and after her internship opened a general practice in a small community in upper New York State, said that her practice grew to full size almost as soon as she set it up, and she had

[16] Josephine J. Williams, "The professional status of women in medicine" (unpublished Ph.D. dissertation, Department of Sociology, University of Chicago, 1949), p. 105.

to wait far less for patients than her white classmates. (Although her practice remained predominately Negro, she received more white patients as she went on.) In fact, it became so overpoweringly large that on the birth of her third child she decided to give it up altogether, switching to a full-time position at a clinic, which still left most of her evenings free.

Due to social factors within the Negro community, few physicians receive certification as specialists: for many, the expense and length of training demanded is too great, and even with certification there is little opportunity for a financially rewarding practice as a specialist. Negro general practitioners are said to refer their patients to a white specialist when one is needed, while the most specialized of Negro physicians receive large numbers of Negro patients requiring general medical help.[17] Recently, a new problem has arisen because of the disproportionate number of highly trained Negro women to Negro men (a problem which extends to finding mates as well). At a Conference on Negroes for Medicine held by the Josiah Macy, Jr., Foundation in the spring of 1967, participants from the Negro community took the position that in the future, preference should be given to aid Negro men seeking a medical education, rather than women, until a balance is established.

As with Negroes who often become overloaded with general practice from their own communities, many women physicians in private practice report that a large segment of their patients are women. One woman internist who devoted more than 60 hours per week to her practice, found that her office was filled with young girls who were referred to her by their friends for gynecological work. She explained that many girls, particularly if they are not married, are uncomfortable about asking about birth control, and they feel that a woman physician will not censure them or probe around unnecessarily as a man might. Women in their forties and fifties also sought out the internist. She explained this as follows:

---

[17] "Negro physicians and other Negro health personnel," A reseacrh agenda prepared by the Health Resource Study Center, University of Washington Medical School, 1966.

"When they were younger, they enjoyed visiting a male doctor, but now they're becoming self-conscious about their bodies getting ugly, and they'd rather have a woman examine them." She also got calls from middle-aged women who came to her because they were virgins and felt shy or humiliated when being examined by a man.

Whatever reluctance may exist among the public to consulting a woman physician, enough patients are available to keep the most ambitious woman busy, and many women in private practice have switched to a salaried position because they find themselves unable to control the amount of time demanded by patients. The chart below gives a run-down of the principal types of employment of a national sample of men and women doctors practicing in 1964. These statistics do not reflect the actual proportions of women to men in the various fields, since the sample taken here is roughly

TABLE 10–2.   CLASSIFICATION BY PRINCIPAL EMPLOYER
as REPORTED TO A.M.A.

Principal employer	Women No. (per cent)		Men No. (per cent)	
Research institutions excluding hospitals	12	0.9	6	0.4
Clinic or physician employer	60	4.5	68	4.3
Medical school or parent university	90	6.7	72	4.5
Other educational institution	30	2.2	6	0.4
Federal government				
Military (Air Force, Army, Navy)	5	0.4	36	2.3
U.S. Public Health Service	6	0.5	12	0.8
Veterans Administration	39	2.9	34	2.1
Other	8	0.6	2	0.1
Non-federal				
Public Health Department	97	7.3	22	1.4
Hospitals	176	13.2	100	6.3
Pharmaceutical and other industries	13	0.9	19	1.2
Self-employed	642	48.1	1,192	75.3
No data	158	11.8	15	0.9
Totals	1,336	100.0	1,584	100.0

Source: Lee Powers, Harry Wiesenfelder, and Rexford C. Parmelee, "Practice patterns of women and men physicians," Preliminary Report (October, 1966), Table 26.

equal for both sexes, while only about one in twelve physicians in the United States is a woman. But it does show that a far higher percentage of women than men enter salaried positions, particularly in non-government institutions.

Men are under-represented in these areas partly because salaried jobs are, in general, not as financially remunerative as even a private practice with limited hours would be. This may help to account for the fact that the median income for women working 2,000 hours or more in 1964 was $16,132, while the median income for men working 2,000 or more hours was $25,879. Those women who worked less than 2,000 hours during the year earned $8,635 —only half of the men's median earnings of $19,791 for approximately the same number of hours.[18] In the salaried positions themselves—civil service or otherwise—it is common knowledge that some of the highest-paying jobs are associated with men, and that the silent requirement is that the candidate be male.

Professional advancement in the medical world is one area where those women who claim prejudice have the facts on their side. Women do not advance in staff positions in the medical schools, hospitals, or other institutions at the same rate as men. Out of 1,047 department chairmen in 78 U.S. medical schools, only 13 are women; there are only 105 women with the rank of professor, as compared to 2,554 men. At the lower end of the academic ranks, however, women take up far more than their 6 per cent of the total medical population: 770 women are instructors and 2,132 men hold the same rank; 104 women are senior instructors, while 263 senior instructors are men.[19]

An example of the artificiality of few women being in top administrative positions and the ease with which this can be remedied was provided by the Veterans Administration. Between 1958 and 1966, only six women—in contrast to 500 men—attended the

[18] Powers, Wiesenfelder, and Parmelee, "Practice patterns of women and men physicians" (1966), Table 19.
[19] "Faculty rank by sex and age for 78 of the U.S. medical schools in operation in 1965–66 academic year." *Faculty Roster,* Association of American Medical Colleges, 1966.

management institution for chiefs of staff of the 165 V.A. hospitals throughout the country. In 1966, when an official memorandum was distributed to all department and staff office heads to the effect that "more V.A. women should be given the benefit of high level management training," there was a sudden influx of the appointment of women physicians to this program: the next session included 11 women among 24 top-management participants. Many of the women had been in secondary positions, some of them assuming that the top was purely a "man's world," particularly since it was an organization linked to the military establishment.[20]

One very important reason why women doctors do not demand all that they might in the work situation—and this includes leaves, referrals, and society membership, as well as promotions—is that they often feel insecure about their bargaining power. In one case, a woman may feel that a promotion is in order, but knows that a man in a similar position has worked full-time since he entered the institution, while she had worked only three-quarters of the time for several years when her children were young. In another case, the woman knows that even if she demanded it, her request would carry little weight: because of her husband's job and her children's school, she is tied to this particular locale, and she cannot threaten her superiors with leaving for an institution somewhere else, forcing them to match the offer.

In addition, many women with young children are unsure of how much more they can take on, and often remain at a job below their aspirations rather than push for a work-load which they are not quite certain they could accomplish comfortably and in good form. A physician in public health said she had simply decided that "Some people are chiefs and some are Indians," and that she would be an Indian as long as her children were young. But, when a job fell into her lap to organize a program she did not refuse it and found after an initial adjustment that she could manage both ends of her responsibilities surprisingly well.

[20] Elizabeth Shilton, "Woman heads Chicago V.A. hospital," *Washington Post,* May 20, 1966, p. B–2.

XI

CONCLUSION

It has been my intention in this book to communicate what it is like to be a woman in medicine in the United States. Summarizing the contradictory and ambiguous impressions of women physicians would be an impossible task, and in a stream of generalizations the small, individual realities that I have tried to convey in the previous pages would be lost. These have taken precedence over any single thesis: the present book should not be regarded as an attempt to present "the case for women doctors," or to sell them to the public or medical administrators—although if such aims have been accomplished along the way that is all to the good.

Nevertheless, a few points may be made in this conclusion to add to the suggestions for improvements—such as increased scholarship aid to medical students, more flexible scheduling during the training years, and child-care tax deductions—which have been scattered throughout the book. Women today are admitted into medicine in token numbers. The percentage may increase in the next ten years, since specialties such as psychiatry, pediatrics, and public health which have traditionally attracted women are reporting serious shortages, and perhaps due to the former, some measures have been taken to make training more feasible for the married woman. However, although the number of women in medicine should definitely be increased from the present low 6 to 8 per cent, it would be pointless to demand that medical schools increase the proportion of women to 20 per cent, 30 per cent, or any other cut-off figure that would begin to represent their numbers in the general population. As it now stands, the percentage of women admitted is the same as the percentage who apply each year, and admitting a larger proportion of applicants might mean taking inferior candidates. Until young girls receive a different set of goals for their adult lives, it is unlikely that substantially more than are presently applying will graduate from college with their desire to enter medicine intact. What seems necessary is that the national climate of opinion concerning sexual roles be changed so that many more high-caliber women will, of their own choice, decide to become doctors and will squeeze their way into the medical world.

In the United States, a country meek about taking committed action to resolve its social problems, it may require time for the social climate to become conducive to women entering medicine or other professions. Numerous psychological and sociological studies have established that American girls are dissuaded from showing independence and intellectual originality, and are instead encouraged to become homemakers who adapt to situations and live through the achievement of their husbands and children. Altering the traditional male and female roles so that the members of both sexes can achieve their fullest potential will necessitate change on all levels, from rewriting children's books to include the working mommy as well as daddy, to a shift in the educational curriculum away from home-arts for girls. An emphasis in the mass media on the contributions of women professionals is another of the host of steps to be taken which may seem minor at first, but are actually indispensable in changing a child's approach to life.

The present women physicians are in many ways guinea pigs for future generations, sometimes performing this function happily, and at other times grudgingly. Many are trying to find out for themselves whether it is possible to combine the satisfactions that are traditionally feminine with the fulfillments of an engrossing, all-encompassing profession like medicine. Little is being done by American society, however, to make their double burden any lighter. Becoming a professional woman still means, in most instances, taking on the jobs of two people instead of one. And because of the pressures on women at this stage to prove that they are worthy of being admitted into the professional world, they are often reluctant to accept concessions which might help them to perform better their dual jobs. Unless it can become more commonplace for a woman to enter medicine or any other "masculine" field, there is little likelihood that this reluctance will lessen, or that in consequence a larger number of women will seek to gain entrance.

The circle is self-perpetuating, although by no means hopeless. Women do offer an untapped source of talent; they can help to fill both a quantitative and a qualitative need for physicians. In addition, medicine in the United States is coming into an era in which large amounts of overhauling and restructuring may be necessary. There are indications that the directions of proposed reform could turn it into a profession which is, incidentally, more congenial and inviting to women practitioners.

It may also be of slight consolation to know that even those countries most advanced in their use of womanpower have not wholly solved the problem of easing the woman's double burden. The socialistic governments have yet to produce sufficient nurseries and crèches for the children of their working women, nor have they organized efficient squadrons of domestic help. But in the meantime, the working women in these countries have come to regard their careers as indispensable sources of stimulation and accomplishment, and have preferred to work at both jobs rather than to give up their professional interests.

What may make the prospect of becoming a physician worthwhile for the young woman is not necessarily the financial gain or guaranteed security—although these may be pleasant dividends. It is the enrichment of her life, the full use of her gifts, the sense of self-expansion which cannot be dismissed easily, even after she considers the obstacles it may bring. Perhaps this enrichment is the line of attack which those seeking more women in medicine should take.

APPENDIX

APPENDIX I

Women in Medicine in the United States, 1905–65

Year	Women students	Percentage of all students	Women graduates	Percentage of all graduates
1905	1,073	4.1	219	4.0
1910	907	4.0	116	2.6
1915	592	4.0	92	2.6
1920	818	5.8	122	4.0
1925	910	5.0	204	5.1
1926	935	5.0	212	5.4
1927	964	4.9	189	4.7
1928	929	4.5	207	4.9
1929	925	4.4	214	4.8
1930	955	4.4	204	4.5
1931	990	4.5	217	4.6
1932	955	4.3	208	4.2
1933	1,056	4.7	214	4.4
1934	1,020	4.5	211	4.2
1935	1,077	4.7	207	4.1
1936	1,133	5.0	246	4.7
1937	1,113	5.1	238	4.4
1938	1,161	5.4	237	4.6
1939	1,144	5.4	260	5.1
1940	1,145	5.4	253	5.0
1941	1,146	5.4	280	5.3
1942	1,164	5.3	279	5.4
1943	1,150	5.1	241	4.6
1944	1,176	5.0	239	4.7
1944 (2d sess.)	1,141	4.6	252	4.9
1945	1,352	5.6	262	5.1
1946	1,868	8.0	242	4.2
1947[1]	2,183	9.1	342	5.4
1948	2,159	9.5	392	7.1
1949	2,100	8.9	612	12.1
1950	1,806	7.2	595	10.7
1951	1,564	5.9	468	7.6
1952	1,471	5.4	351	5.7
1953	1,463	5.3	363	5.5
1954	1,502	5.3	360	5.2
1955	1,537	5.4	345	4.9
1956	1,573	5.5	340	5.0
1957	1,646	5.7	330	5.0
1958	1,644	5.6	355	5.1
1959	—	—	370	5.4
1960	1,710	6.0	405	5.7
1961	1,745	5.8	354	5.3
1962	1,955	6.3	391	5.8
1963	2,081	6.7	405	5.9
1964	2,244	7.0	449	6.5
1965	2,503	7.7	503	7.3

Note: [1] Includes additional classes.
Source: JAMA Education Number.

APPENDIX II

Acceptance Data on Men and Women Applicants for Selected Years[1]

Year	Men			Women			Women as per cent of total acceptances
	Number Applicants	Number Accepted	Per cent Accepted	Number Applicants	Number Accepted	Per cent Accepted	
1929–30	13,174	6,720	51.0	481	315	65.5	4.5
1935–36	12,051	6,521	54.1	689	379	55.0	5.5
1940–41	11,269	6,025	53.5	585	303	51.8	4.8
1950–51	21,049	6,869	32.6	1,231	385	31.3	5.3
1955–56	13,935	7,465	53.6	1,002	504	50.3	6.3
1960–61	13,353	7,960	59.6	1,044	600	57.5	7.0
1961–62	13,215	7,946	60.1	1,166	736	63.2	8.5
1962–63	14,646	8,242	56.3	1,201	717	59.7	8.0
1963–64	16,236	8,305	51.2	1,432	758	52.9	8.4
1964–65	17,437	8,219	47.1	1,731	824	47.6	9.1

Note: [1] Earlier data are presented at five-year intervals where available.

Source: Education numbers of the JAMA for appropriate years.

APPENDIX III

(A) Dropout Trends by Sex, 1949–58 Entrants[1]

Entering year	Total entrants		Per cent active dropouts		Per cent non-active dropouts		Per cent total dropouts	
	Men	Women	Men	Women	Men	Women	Men	Women
1949	6,731	404	4.40	4.70	3.48	7.43	7.87	12.13
1950	6,798	377	3.60	3.98	2.84	6.37	6.44	10.34
1951	7,032	403	4.11	7.98	2.45	7.44	6.56	15.38
1952	7,046	409	4.64	6.11	2.92	8.07	7.56	14.18
1953	6,980	434	4.80	7.14	3.17	10.83	7.97	17.97
1954	7,051	439	4.84	9.34	3.43	9.34	8.27	18.68
1955	7,172	452	5.17	7.96	3.49	10.40	8.66	18.36
1956	7,396	497	5.76	8.05	3.39	6.04	9.15	14.08
1957	7,434	448	5.73	9.38	4.02	8.93	9.75	18.30
1958	7,500	450	6.47	7.78	3.71	6.89	10.17	14.67
Total	71,140	4,313	4.98	7.33	3.30	8.18	8.28	15.51

(B) Class Year of 1961–62 Female Respondents to Attrition Study Questionnaires

Progress group	Fresh.	Soph.	Jr.	Sr.	Not in school, 61–62	Total
Regular	37	27	30	27	1	122
Repeater	6	8	—	—	—	14[2]
Academic dropout	15	4	1	—	—	20[2]
Non-academic dropout	24	5	2	—	—	31
Total	82	44	33	27	1	187

Notes: [1] Summarized at the request of Carol Lopate, Josiah Macy, Jr. Foundation.
 [2] These figures will probably be revised to read: 12 repeaters and 22 academic dropouts.

Source: Table 1–A of Data Book No. 1, Association of American Medical Colleges.

APPENDIX IV

(A) Detailed Occupation of the Experienced Civilian Labor Force
and of the Employed, by Sex—1960 and 1950

PHYSICIANS AND SURGEONS

State	1960				1950			
	Experienced civilian labor force		Employed		Experienced civilian labor force		Employed	
	male	female	male	female	male	female	male	female
Alabama	2,165	105	2,165	105	2,036	95	2,036	94
Alaska	155	27	155	27	73	7	73	7
Arizona	1,386	102	1,382	102	834	43	833	42
Arkansas	1,440	72	1,424	72	1,480	48	1,479	48
California	22,569	2,066	22,494	2,038	15,411	1,414	15,363	1,399
Colorado	2,439	150	2,431	146	1,843	106	1,841	105
Connecticut	3,799	247	3,791	247	3,033	219	3,030	217
Delaware	549	43	549	43	423	22	423	22
District of Columbia	1,524	222	1,516	222	1,764	194	1,764	193
Florida	5,432	270	5,413	270	2,840	112	2,838	111
Georgia	3,465	185	3,465	185	2,728	127	2,728	127
Hawaii	631	84	627	84	464	31	462	31
Idaho	537	16	537	16	463	20	463	19
Illinois	11,949	959	11,908	955	11,670	831	11,649	827
Indiana	4,283	131	4,275	131	3,882	177	3,881	176
Iowa	2,788	167	2,788	167	2,670	125	2,668	124
Kansas	2,595	147	2,587	147	2,159	130	2,159	130
Kentucky	2,553	137	2,545	137	2,351	94	2,350	94
Louisiana	3,203	199	3,195	199	2,842	163	2,838	163
Maine	834	54	829	50	927	35	926	34
Maryland	4,788	417	4,779	414	3,599	290	3,598	290
Massachusetts	8,284	672	8,263	660	7,757	585	7,744	583
Michigan	9,095	505	9,068	493	6,874	357	6,860	352
Minnesota	4,434	273	4,425	269	3,799	233	3,791	231
Mississippi	1,418	60	1,418	56	1,332	35	1,332	35
Missouri	4,827	364	4,823	356	4,828	275	4,824	273
Montana	566	19	558	19	532	30	531	30
Nebraska	1,573	66	1,569	63	1,407	61	1,406	61
Nevada	348	20	348	20	200	4	200	4

(A) Detailed Occupation of the Experienced Civilian Labor Force and of the Employed, by Sex—1960 and 1950

PHYSICIANS AND SURGEONS

	1960				1950			
State	Experienced civilian labor force		Employed		Experienced civilian labor force		Employed	
	male	female	male	female	male	female	male	female
New Hampshire	591	33	591	33	598	47	597	47
New Jersey	8,063	669	8,047	661	6,630	425	6,616	422
New Mexico	777	50	773	50	531	34	530	34
New York	29,595	3,121	29,510	3,093	28,269	2,359	28,175	2,345
North Carolina	3,722	259	3,711	259	2,939	163	2,934	163
North Dakota	490	20	486	20	456	14	456	14
Ohio	11,404	634	11,383	625	9,227	526	9,219	522
Oklahoma	2,374	162	2,374	158	2,071	91	2,070	91
Oregon	2,121	94	2,121	94	1,716	118	1,712	117
Pennsylvania	14,374	1,111	14,357	1,102	13,090	909	13,071	906
Rhode Island	1,078	49	1,074	49	931	61	928	61
South Carolina	1,667	98	1,667	98	1,409	43	1,408	43
South Dakota	493	35	493	35	505	29	503	29
Tennessee	3,658	212	3,654	212	2,941	138	2,940	138
Texas	9,177	503	9,152	495	7,280	366	7,275	365
Utah	1,009	41	1,009	41	769	28	768	28
Vermont	528	65	524	65	468	35	468	33
Virginia	4,210	257	4,210	257	3,104	177	3,103	175
Washington	3,253	196	3,253	196	2,623	132	2,621	131
West Virginia	1,634	90	1,630	83	1,646	57	1,646	56
Wisconsin	3,833	183	3,829	183	3,406	204	3,400	204
Wyoming	238	11	238	11	239	6	238	6

Source: U.S. Bureau of Census, U.S. Census of Population, 1960 (Washington: U.S. Government Printing Office, 1962).

(B) Women Physicians and Surgeons, December, 1965

State	No.	State	No.
Alabama	110	Nevada	9
Alaska	25	New Hampshire	74
Arizona	99	New Jersey	658
Arkansas	63	New Mexico	61
California	2,452	New York	3,792
Canal Zone	7	North Carolina	254
Colorado	182	North Dakota	14
Connecticut	357	Ohio	849
Delaware	52	Oklahoma	120
District of Columbia	388	Oregon	134
Florida	368	Pennsylvania	1,306
Georgia	214	Puerto Rico	153
Hawaii	71	Rhode Island	84
Idaho	17	South Carolina	71
Illinois	1,134	South Dakota	26
Indiana	223	Tennessee	208
Iowa	132	Texas	604
Kansas	136	Utah	50
Kentucky	142	Vermont	50
Lousiana	235	Virginia	287
Maine	59	Virgin Islands	5
Maryland	558	Washington	263
Massachusetts	842	West Virginia	77
Michigan	623	Wisconsin	236
Minnesota	252	Wyoming	6
Mississippi	67	Foreign, including Canada	280
Missouri	278	Others	363
Montana	21		
Nebraska	40	Total	19,181

Source: American Medical Women's Association, Inc.

APPENDIX V

Faculty Rank by Sex and Age for 78 of the U.S. Medical Schools
in Operation in 1965–66 Academic Years[1]

	Total all ages	Less than 30	30–39	40–49	50–59	60 and over	No response
Female							
Department Chairman	13	—	2	1	5	4	1
Professor	105	3	6	20	43	25	8
Associate Professor	356	2	45	158	101	32	18
Assistant Professor	693	16	245	257	105	28	42
Senior Instructor	104	9	39	31	17	5	3
Instructor	770	103	314	172	85	19	77
Other titles or title unknown	71	10	7	29	14	—	11
Subtotal	2,112	143	658	668	370	113	160
Male							
Department Chairman	1,034	5	68	388	388	154	31
Professor	2,554	39	186	1,006	899	335	89
Associate Professor	3,499	16	889	1,911	469	86	128
Assistant Professor	4,774	81	2,993	1,265	179	30	226
Senior Instructor	263	11	164	64	14	1	9
Instructor	2,132	153	1,497	252	57	9	164
Other titles or title unknown	266	15	96	79	51	18	7
Subtotal	14,522	320	5,893	4,965	2,057	633	654

	Department Chairman	Professor	Associate Professor	Assistant Professor	Senior Instructor	Instructor	Other titles or title unknown	Total
No response to sex	1	2	10	46	6	44	3	112
Total men and women	1,047	2,659	3,855	5,467	367	2,902	337	16,634
Total	1,048	2,661	3,865	5,513	373	2,946	340	16,746

[1] "Faculty rank by sex and age for 78 of the U.S. medical schools in operation in 1965–66 academic year." *Faculty Roster* (Association of American Medical Colleges, 1966).

INDEX

Designed by Edward King

*Composed in Fairfield with Perpetua display
by Monotype Composition Co. Inc.*

*Printed offset by Universal Lithographers, Inc.
on P&S R*

*Bound by L. H. Jenkins in Holliston Zeppelin with
printed Multicolor endpapers*

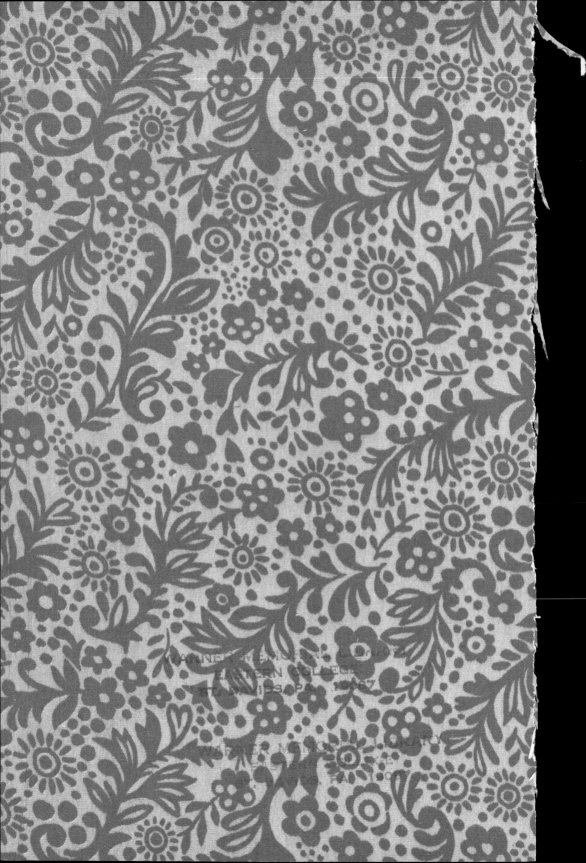